Laparoscopic Colon Surgery

Gregory Kouraklis
Eugenia (Jenny) Matsiota
Editors

Laparoscopic Colon Surgery

Milestones, Education, & Best Practice

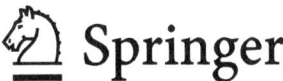 Springer

Editors
Gregory Kouraklis
Department of Propaedeutic Surgery
School of Medicine at the National and
Kapodistrian University of Athens
Athens
Greece

Eugenia (Jenny) Matsiota
Public Administration and Liberal Arts
Hankuk University of Foreign Studies
Seoul
Korea (Republic of)

ISBN 978-3-030-56727-9   ISBN 978-3-030-56728-6   (eBook)
https://doi.org/10.1007/978-3-030-56728-6

This Springer imprint is published by the registered company Springer Nature Switzerland AG
The registered company address is: Gewerbestrasse 11, 6330 Cham, Switzerland

Foreword

I am delighted to write the foreword for the first edition of the book *Laparoscopic Colon Surgery: Milestones, Education, & Best Practice*. I hold high respect for the editors of this book whose diversity, knowledge, and high caliber skills, each one in their field of expertise, make an astonishing combination for producing a succinct manuscript that can showcase the milestones, education, and best practices of laparoscopic colon surgery.

There are still prevailing difficulties in endorsing the laparoscopic technique in colon surgery. Although conventional laparoscopic procedures have a long history and practice, laparoscopic colon surgery does not constitute the first choice for most surgeons who would prefer open surgery despite sufficient clinical evidence showing that laparoscopic technique in colon treatment has equal clinical results as open surgery but is also a more efficient technique for the healthcare system with fewer operating hours, fewer days of hospitalization, quicker recovery, and less pain and trauma for the patient.

I have been an advocate of laparoscopic colon surgery almost since the beginning of my career having a big record of cases of both benign and malignant diseases. Through this vast experience I have succeeded to offer my patients the benefits of a treatment that renders better quality of care and recovery. I also had the pleasure and the privilege to educate and train novice surgeons in laparoscopic colon surgery and guide them through the fundamental process of evaluating and selecting the right patients, understand the anatomical challenges, and plan a surgery accordingly.

This book will give readers the opportunity to understand the importance of properly organizing and evaluating each step in a well-designed laparoscopic colon surgery to achieve optimal results, not only for the patients but also for the healthcare system and its stakeholders. In contemporary healthcare organizations, cost-effective treatment is a mandate. This book sheds plenty of light on many aspects and considerations of laparoscopic colon surgery that can contribute to cost-effectiveness. It highlights aspects of proper instrument selection, effective training, effective anesthesia and surgical planning, accurate management of complications, and adequate post-surgical follow-up. It advances knowledge by including a chapter that elaborates on the characteristics, benefits, and concerns of robotic surgery in colon cancer.

The editors of this book have made an excellent choice in putting together the thematic chapters and therefore information that can enhance knowledge and understanding, which can help novice or experienced surgeons to decide on career advancement and specialization. Moreover, the book triggers thinking about educational curricula and training methods that can be used to enhance the employment of laparoscopic colon surgery instead of open surgery. The use of simulators, in addition to traditional methods of training, is extensively discussed encouraging academicians to consider a paradigm shift in surgical training that can be more effective and efficient, offering optimal results for patients but also for the healthcare organizations and the quality of care they pursue to offer.

This book represents a systematic attempt to explain the benefits of laparoscopic colon surgery for patients, surgeons, surgical educators, and administrators.

September 10, 2020

Konstantinos M. Konstantinidis
Department of General Bariatric,
Laparoscopic and Robotic Surgery
Athens Medical Center
Athens, Greece

Ohio State University
Columbus, OH, USA

American College of Surgeons,
Greek Chapter (ACS-GC)
Chicago, IL, USA

Clinical Robotic Surgery
Association, (CRSA)
Chicago, IL, USA

International Board of Directors,
Society of Robotic Surgery, (SRS)
East Dundee, IL, USA

Preface

This book represents an effort to give the reader a succinct understanding of laparoscopic colon surgery (LCS). It is for both experienced and novice surgeons. The authors aspire to offer an understanding of the main advantages, concerns, and areas for improvement of LCS. Throughout the book, emphasis is placed in the need for dedicated training and education that can expand the endorsement of LCS, offering better results to the patients and improving the quality of care offered.

What is very distinct in this book is that not all authors are surgeons or medical doctors. The emphasis on safety, education, quality of care, and cost of healthcare has allowed diverse healthcare practitioners and scholars to contribute to this book, sharing their ideas, opinions, and suggestions for the improvement and hopefully the broader acceptance of LCS treatment.

The endeavor in this first edition is to fend off confusion and anxiety between LCS and open colon surgery. By reading this book, surgeons should be able to identify the criteria that can lead their choices for the most suitable surgical treatment, and healthcare decision-makers can get an understanding of the training needs of their institutions, as well as the wise allocation of resources that can potentially offer cost-effective solutions to enhance competitiveness and sustainability.

This book assumes familiarity with basic healthcare terms and basic knowledge of surgical practices. It is not meant to stand alone but in conjunction with other books of general laparoscopy and surgical treatment.

Finally, the editors and the notable authors of this book wish that this work can trigger new thoughts about best surgical practices that will result from adequate and continuous learning and training. The ultimate goals are to enhance quality of care, patient satisfaction, and cost-containment; critical factors of healthcare that decision-makers in any institution should consider to stay abreast with the needs and requirements of contemporary systems.

Athens, Greece   Gregory Kouraklis
Seoul, Republic of Korea   Eugenia (Jenny) Matsiota

Contents

Contributors

Chrysanthi Aggeli Third Department of Surgery, General Hospital of Athens "G. Gennimatas", Athens, Greece

George Bagias 1st Propaedeutic Surgical Department, Hippokration Hospital, University of Athens, Athens, Greece

Konstantinos Bramis Aretaieio Hospital of Athens, National and Kapodistrian University of Athens, Athens, Greece

D. Daniel León CDD Las Mercedes, Caracas, Venezuela

Phillip L. Davidson, PhD Doctoral Program Faculty for Business Management in Organizational Leadership and IST, University of Phoenix, College of Doctoral Studies, Phoenix, AZ, USA

Amalia Douma Department of Anaesthesiology, General Hospital of Athens "G. Gennimatas", Athens, Greece

Zoi Garoufalia Faculty of Medicine, 2nd Propedeutic Surgical Department, Laiko General Hospital, National and Kapodistrian University of Athens, Athens, Greece

Ifigeneia Grigoriadou Department of Anaesthesiology, General Hospital of Athens "G. Gennimatas", Athens, Greece

Ioannis D. Kostakis Faculty of Medicine, 2nd Propedeutic Surgical Department, Laiko General Hospital, National and Kapodistrian University of Athens, Athens, Greece

Gregory Kouraklis Department of Propaedeutic Surgery, School of Medicine at the National and Kapodistrian University of Athens, Athens, Greece

Ioannis Makris Professor Emeritus (Retired), School of Medicine, Aristotle University of Thessaloniki, Thessaloniki, Greece

Dimitrios Mantas Faculty of Medicine, 2nd Propedeutic Surgical Department, Laiko General Hospital, National and Kapodistrian University of Athens, Athens, Greece

Eugenia (Jenny) Matsiota Visiting Professor, Public Administration and Liberal Arts, Hankuk University of Foreign Studies, Seoul, Republic of Korea

Constantinos S. Mavrantonis, MD, PhD, FACS 6th Department of Surgery— SRC Center of Excellence for Colorectal Surgery, Hygeia Hospital, Athens, Greece

Chairman, NoDE Institute, Athens, Greece

Adamantios Michalinos Department of Anatomy, Faculty of Medicine, European University of Cyprus, Nicosia, Cyprus

Petros Mirilas 'Aghia Sophia' Children's Hospital, Athens, Greece

University Paris XIII- Léonard de Vinci, Courbevoie, France

Surgical Anatomy & Technique, Emory University, Atlanta, GA, USA

Alexander-Michael Nixon Third Department of Surgery, General Hospital of Athens "G. Gennimatas", Athens, Greece

Sotirios George Panousopoulos, MD, PhD 6th Department of Surgery—SRC Center of Excellence for Colorectal Surgery, Hygeia Hospital, Athens, Greece

Director, Simulation Center—NoDE Institute, Athens, Greece

Vasileios Papaziogas Director of 2nd Surgery Clinic of AUTH, Professor of Surgery AUTH, School of Medicine, Aristotle University of Thessaloniki, Thessaloniki, Greece

University of Munich, Munich, Germany

George P. Skandalakis Department of Anatomy, Faculty of Medicine, National and Kapodistrian University of Athens, Athens, Greece

Panayiotis N. Skandalakis Anatomy and Surgical Anatomy, National and Kapodistrian University of Athens, Athens, Greece

Theodore G. Troupis Department of Anatomy, Faculty of Medicine, National and Kapodistrian University of Athens, Athens, Greece

A. Wilson Mourad CDD Las Mercedes, Caracas, Venezuela

Georgios N. Zografos Third Department of Surgery, General Hospital of Athens "G. Gennimatas", Athens, Greece

Introduction

The introduction of laparoscopy into the field of general surgery has been a revelation, and it is the single most important change in surgical technique of the past decades. It has turned the way of thinking in surgery. The adage *"big surgeon, big wounds"* no longer applies and is replaced by a collective awareness that the approach in surgery must be as minimal as possible. Laparoscopic cholecystectomy is the most common laparoscopic surgical procedure. On the contrary, the laparoscopic surgical technique is not widely accepted when it comes to laparoscopic colectomy.

Laparoscopic colectomy is a minimal invasive technique that has limited application until today. Although 26 years have passed since the first laparoscopic colectomy, it is still not the first choice. Surgeons prefer the open colectomy surgical technique although clinical studies support that the outcomes of both open and laparoscopic techniques are the same in benign and malignant tumors, with the laparoscopic technique surpassing the open colectomy because it causes less trauma, offers more patient comfort, faster postoperative recovery with earlier return to daily activities, and fewer days of hospitalization. Nevertheless, in the United States, surgeons treat one third of colectomy cases with open surgery. Even when surgeons start the surgery with laparoscopy, the conversion rate to open surgery remains high. The main reason for the limited application of laparoscopic colectomy is the anatomical difficulties of the colon and the associated stiff learning curve.

Preoperative evaluation and adequate preparation of patients, thorough study of the patients' physiology, good anatomic knowledge, and the use of proper surgical instruments and techniques are important factors contributing to a successful laparoscopic colectomy with low conversion rates. Of course, the quality and adequacy of training and the continuous education surgeon should be receiving are of utmost importance. Many scholars support that laparoscopic colectomy is more effective when performed in high-volume hospitals, where the large number of cases allow quicker progress in the learning curve. Of significant concern in laparoscopic colon surgery is the time needed to complete the surgery in the operating room, which is associated with intra- and postoperative complications and high cost. To be able to reduce the operating time, skills need to be improved through continuous practice. Training on cadavers but especially on simulators is a safe and cost-effective alternative for both high-volume and lower-volume hospitals, with the last having an even greater need for following alternative, but effective, methods of surgical training like the training on simulators. Technological advancements on simulators have come out with software programs that give such haptic feedback and tactile sensation that very closely simulate the reality.

As robotic surgery is advancing, it also starts finding a place in laparoscopic colon surgery. Robotic colon surgical procedures are mainly performed in teaching hospitals and metropolitan areas, and although there is still a long way to prove its effectiveness and necessity, laparoscopic colon surgery appears to be promising, offering some benefits such as faster recovery of the bowel function and lower risk of incisional hernia. Still training and experience are crucial parameters for a successful robotic operation.

Fast-track management is another significant process described in this book, which can offer better quality of care and earlier discharge and ultimately decrease cost. Fast-track aims personalized treatment to improve recovery and achieve a reduction in the postoperative length of stay. Personalized treatment requires the cooperation of a multidisciplinary team, physicians who can study patients case by case and closely cooperate to maintain optimum cardiovascular, pulmonary, gastrointestinal, neurological, and humoral functions. Fast-track concerns rigorous preoperative and postoperative management. The preoperative care is crucial because it can better prepare patients for the laparoscopic colorectal surgery, helping both patients and surgeons to avoid intraoperative complications. Postoperative analgesia avoidance of nasogastric tubes and drains, early oral fluid intake, and early mobilization contribute to early recovery, which results in better quality of care, early discharge (2–3 days quicker than laparoscopic colectomy surgery without fast-track management), and thus less cost for the healthcare system.

The increase in colon cancer cases, the more informed and demanding patients, and the contemporary healthcare trends for quality of care and cost-containment triggered the idea of creating a book specifically about laparoscopic colectomy. This book addresses mainly colon tumors. Reference to rectal tumors is limited because the available experience with laparoscopic surgery for rectal cancer is scarce and because the treatment of rectal cancer differs from that of colon cancer in many respects. The aim of the book is to assess laparoscopic practice surgery as curative treatment for colon cancer and to shed light on laparoscopic colectomy learning. The effort is to offer comprehensive and succinct information about laparoscopic colectomy to any surgeon, experienced or beginner, who considers choosing laparoscopic colectomy as a surgical technique.

Hyperspecialization has only recently been introduced into surgical training at an early stage. From their third year of residency, surgeons in training should exclusively be tutored in one of the four main directions in general surgery, i.e., oncologic, gastrointestinal, vascular, or trauma surgery. A main obligation of the gastrointestinal surgeon performing colon surgery should be to obtain sufficient laparoscopic skills. The advanced laparoscopic skills required for minimally invasive colon surgery can only be maintained when the colon surgeon performs laparoscopic surgery in sufficient numbers. This warrants further centralization of laparoscopic treatment of colon cancer.

The objectives of this book are to identify the preferred diagnostic procedures and the correct selection of patients and describe the right surgical techniques for laparoscopic resection of colon cancer. Also, the book aims to assess quality and effectiveness of care in terms of morbidity, hospital stay, cost, and recovery, to delineate the standards and optimal practices for laparoscopic colon cancer surgery, as well as to provide recommendation statements that reflect what is known and what constitutes good practice. The future of surgical colon treatment belongs to minimal invasive techniques, better aesthetic results, more comfort for the patient, less complications, and fewer days of hospitalization.

Eugenia (Jenny) Matsiota

Eugenia (Jenny) Matsiota and Phillip L. Davidson

1.1   Introduction

The term "laparoscopic surgery" refers to a class of minimally invasive surgeries [1]. There are many subsets under this term such as laparoscopic cholecystectomy, appendectomy, hysterectomy, colon, and colorectal surgery. "Laparoscopic surgery" is also referred as minimally invasive surgery (MIS) and sometimes the two terms are used interchangeably. For clarification, MIS is typically used to refer to *any* procedure that minimizes the invasiveness of surgery and includes such practices as arthroscopy, robotic surgery, head and neck, gynecological, urological, and other endoscopic surgical procedures. The challenge to the surgeon revolves around what the physician can see, do, and treat, how visualization is brought about, and how accessible the human organ is with less traumatic interventions. Open surgery, the opposite of MIS, requires larger incisions to allow the surgeon to see and treat the affected organ [2]. Because incisions are larger in open surgery, there is more trauma and blood loss to the patient [3]. One of the primary arguments for MIS is that it is less invasive, where the surgeon limits the size of the trauma to small ports to insert visualization devices, such as an arthroscope, endoscope, or laparoscope, and surgical instruments to perform the surgery [4]. In some cases, like hand-assisted laparoscopy, an additional small incision may be required, which is still much smaller than the incision of an open surgery.

E. (J.) Matsiota
Visiting Professor, Public Administration and Liberal Arts, Hankuk University of Foreign Studies, Seoul, Republic of Korea

P. L. Davidson (✉)
Doctoral Program Faculty for Business Management in Organizational Leadership and IST, University of Phoenix, College of Doctoral Studies, Phoenix, AZ, USA
e-mail: phil.davidson@phoenix.edu

In this chapter, the focus is on MIS, specifically laparoscopic surgery. However, in the "formalized" practice of medicine, defined here as the time from Hippocrates to the present, laparoscopic surgery only appeared a little over 100 years ago [5]. As Harrell and Heniford noted, laparoscopic surgery evolved from numerous technological innovations. This chapter will be used to focus on those innovations and the innovators through medical history, concluding with a brief look at the current status and perhaps a brief peek into the future.

1.2 Definitions

1.2.1 Endoscopy

An examination of the inside of the body through a lighted, flexible or rigid, tube called an endoscope [6]. Typically, an endoscope is introduced into the body through a natural opening, such as the mouth or anus. Endoscopy or endoscope derive from the Greek words ἔνδον (*éndon*) meaning "in" or within, plus σκοπέω (skopeo) meaning "to look at" or examine [7]. Physicians use the endoscope to see internal parts of the body like the throat, esophagus, kidney, and bladder.

1.2.2 Laparoscopy

A process that uses a specialized endoscope inserted through the abdominal wall, specifically for examining or "visualizing" the internal organs. The word derives from the Greek word λαπάρα *(lapara)* which means "flank" or abdomen and σκοπέω *(skopeo)* meaning "to look at" or examine. Laparoscopy concerns the insertion to the human body of an instrument only through the abdominal wall.

1.3 In the Beginning

In the germinal text by Nezhat [8], the author provided an excellent and exhaustive study of endoscopy from its earliest days to the present. For readers who desire that level of detail, the text is highly recommended. In that book, Nezhat breaks the history of endoscopy into many stages. For the sake of brevity, this chapter will be divided into three sections: Ancient, Pre-Modern (19th century), and modern (1900 and forward) times. The dividing lines are somewhat arbitrary, and the focus is more on those pioneers who set the stage for the practice of laparoscopic surgery today rather than arbitrary divisions by year.

1.3.1 Ancient Times

Surgery is an ancient therapeutic method as old as mankind. It has played a significant role throughout the years in the treatment and the healing of wounds. The origin of the word "surgery" comes from the Greek word "chirurgia," which is the combination of two Greek words "cheiros" (hand) and "ergon" (work). In other words, surgery literally means the work of the hand. During the Roman times, the Greek word "chirurgia" became "cirurgie" in Latin, which evolved to "surgerie" in old French, which became "surgery" in the English language.

Surgery is a manual work. The Babylonians and the Assyrians in the ancient Mesopotamian region, today's Iraq, were the first to exercise a primitive kind of surgical treatment. During prehistoric times, people needed to take out from their skin thorns, thistles, pebbles to be able to continue hunting. The oldest recorded surgery is trepanation, which dates to the Neolithic period. The reason people were performing trepanation remains unknown until today [9]. Stunning findings of tools in ancient, prehistoric tombs in Abuser, Upper Egypt such as flint-saws lead to the assumption that cranioplasty was a known method of surgery during that early period [10]. Medicine in ancient Egypt is the oldest documented.

After the pre-historic period, medicine evolved in Persia, India, and Greece [11]. The first recorded doctor to use "macairion" (sword knife) to perform a surgery was Hippocrates, who is considered the father of medicine [12]. The rise of Western Surgery, as it has evolved, has its roots back to ancient Greek times. Archaeologists discovered in a Mycenaean[1] tomb (around 1400BC) surgical instruments like scissors, toothed jaws, needles, chisels, and tongs. The Romans derived most of their medical knowledge from the Greeks, the Egyptians, the Persians, and other people they conquered. Roman surgical instruments were discovered in Pompeii, Italy like scalpels, bone hooks, bone drills, forceps, bone levers, and vaginal and rectal specula [13]. Medical care in ancient Rome was the responsibility of pater familias, the father of the family, who had to possess basic knowledge to offer medical treatment to his family. After Rome conquered Greece, much of the last's medical knowledge influenced Rome. Most of the Roman surgical knowledge was a continuation of the knowledge acquired from the Greeks. Following the ancient Greek doctors, the Romans developed better instruments to be able to perform more demanding surgical operations. Excavations in Pompeii have brought to light more than 13 types of sharp instruments that surgeons of that time were using as sharp knives. Greco-Roman surgical care was advanced and successful in many cases.

Historical findings document the effort of physicians in the ancient world to gain experience in gastroenterology and treat gastrointestinal tract disorders. Hippocrates was the first to perform rectum examination with the use of a speculum [14]. During the classical Greek period, physicians tried to treat the gastrointestinal function through purging cathartics. During the Roman era, Galen focused on the lower gut and advised specific diets and exercise to cope with excrement retention and evacuation disorders. Although, since the very early times, physicians expressed interest and emphasized the treatment of diseases associated with the rectum and the colon, the associated morbidity and mortality rates have always remained high throughout history.

---

[1] Mycenae is an ancient city/polis, an archaeological site today, about 90 km southwest of Athens, Greece, in the Northeastern Peloponnese.

During the Middle Ages, and in most cases, surgeons were not allowed to operate on patients or perform any interventions in the human body. Only a few surgeons in the Western world were not abiding by the rules of the church that was prohibiting any surgical intervention, either in a human or an animal body. Galen was one such doctor, an exceptional and bright example of a doctor who added to the surgical knowledge despite the darkening ideological preaching of Christianity. Galen was a prominent Greek surgeon and philosopher from Pergamon[2] who went to Rome to become a doctor to the emperor. Galen dissected many animals, despite the ban on any dissection, because he believed that knowing the work and structure of the human body was important for any physician and he was trying to gain knowledge from studying the animals' anatomy, the closest possible resemblance to the human anatomy.

Much should be attributed to the Arab doctors of that time, who had no barriers in performing dissections to study the human anatomy. They offered unique, illuminating examples preserving knowledge inherited from old books, saving them from the fire, translating old texts, and advancing the knowledge and practice of surgery. It would not be an exaggeration to support that the preservation of medical knowledge is much owed to the work of the Arab doctors during the dark ages who, when Christianity was suppressing and prohibiting access to knowledge, including the medical legacy of the *paganistic* societies, worked to collect, translate, and save many of the manuscripts.

The goal for most physicians was always to gain a better understanding of what was inside the human body. If that could be done without having to cut open the person, everyone would benefit. As noted, some, such as Hippocrates, used simple tools to look inside the body's natural orifices. The desire to see inside the human body was the motivation behind the search to devise ways to accomplish that feat. However, it is difficult to piece together a history of a specific medical technology, such as endoscopy, from archaeological records and sites. The vocabulary and tools used today must be inferred from bits and pieces of artifacts and incomplete texts.

Most sources attribute the first use of some type of device for internal visualization to Hippocrates (460–375 BCE) [15–18]. According to Nakajima et al., students of the "Kos school of medicine, led by Hippocrates, … described a rectal examination using a speculum remarkably similar to the instruments we use today" (p. 1). Gordon and Magos noted that a speculum for vaginal inspection was found in the ashes of the ruins at Pompeii, the city destroyed by the eruption of Mt. Vesuvius in 70 CE. Other devices and tubes have either been found at archaeological sites or described in ancient manuscripts such as the Babylonian Talmud (500 CE) or seen in paintings and drawings of that time.

Larger and more extensive information becomes available from texts written in the tenth and eleventh centuries. Notable are the voluminous writings of Abu

---

[2] Pergamon was a cultural, powerful, and rich ancient Greek city in Aeolis, Asia Minor. Today is a UNESCO World Heritage Site.

al-Qasim al-Zahrawi (936–1013 CE),[3] whose full name is Abul al-Qasim Khalaf ibn al-Abbas al-Zahrawi, frequently referred to as Albucasis in the west. He will be referred to here as "Al-Zahrawi" [19]. Al-Zahrawi was a prolific pioneer in the field of medicine, and he wrote extensively. He was a Muslim physician, born in Madinat al-Zahra, near Cordova in southern Spain and served as physician to King Al-Hakam-II of Spain. Al-Zahrawi completed a medical encyclopedia of 30 volumes entitled the Al-Tasrif, which included many topics including descriptions reflecting endoscopic techniques. Al-Zahrawi also created a number of proto-endoscopic instruments, although it is unclear as to whether he used any external light source to try to visualize his surgical studies. "For these works alone, Al-Qasim is considered as one of the most important pre-modern founders of endoscopy", p. 8.

While it is unclear as to whether Al-Zahrawi used any type of reflected light in his surgical examinations, Ibn Sînâ (aka "Avicenna," 980–1037 CE), a Persian physician, is credited with being the first to use reflected light to examine body cavities [20]. Avicenna was a highly gifted and productive individual who studied astronomy, math, and medicine among many other topics. He wrote five books entitled the *Al- Qanun fi al-Tibb* ("The Canon of Medicine"). In his text, Avicenna described the use of reflected sunlight and a series of polished mirrors to direct the light for examination of the vulva and cervix of his female patients. The use of any type of light to examine internal anatomy is considered a historical turning point in the history of endoscopy.

It is not the intention to overlook any of the many great visionaries who added to the corpus of knowledge related to the early development of endoscopy and laparoscopy specifically. There are many excellent sources related to specific individuals such as the Italian mathematician Gerolamo Cardano (1501–1576). Cardano, more famous for his book on gambling, also wrote and studied many other topics. He devised a mechanical lantern that changed things forever by using artificial light for examination of the interior of the body. However, as space is limited, for readers who desire greater detail, the text by Nezhat is highly recommended.

1.3.2   Pre-modern Times

There is not much in the way of documentation of archaeological artifacts that suggests significant forward movement in the examination of the internal human body, other than that which has been mentioned. Part of the reason is that for a time there were cultural barriers to dissection. It is not until the eighteenth and nineteenth centuries that significant progress is seen in the internal visualization of the human body. During this period in time, physicians developed the first instruments them inner body visualization.

---

[3] Dates vary for Al-Zahrawi from 936–1013 CE to 980–1037 CE and include sources that combine the two (980–1013 CE). Most use the dates found in this text (980–1037 CE).

One of the first pioneers in the early development of endoscopy was Philipp Bozzini[4] (1773–1809). As noted by Morgenstern [21], Bozzini's family originally came from Italy, but Philipp was born in Germany. Bozzini was an inventor, and the focus here is on his invention, the first "modern endoscope" in 1805 [22]. Bozzini referred to his endoscopic tool as a "Lichtleiter" (light conductor) which involved a concave mirror that reflected light from a candle [23]. Morgenstern describes the Lichtleiter in greater detail stating that the central part of the device looked like a vase, covered in leather. It was a little over 12 in. tall, had an eyepiece for viewing, and light originating from a candle reflected off a mirror.

It is important to understand the situation surrounding Bozzini, as this life was complicated by external circumstances. He worked as a military physician in the imperial army during a time of the War of the Second Coalition (1796–1802) against Napoleon, and his work allowed him to be recognized by important political figures. Unfortunately, the politics surrounding Bozzini and his connection to the imperial army never allowed him to reap the benefits of his work. He died of typhoid fever in 1809 while working with the poor in Frankfort.

Other physician researchers studied and used Bozzini's idea of the Lichtleiter, but it was not until 1865 that Antonin Desormeaux (1815–1894), a French urologist, presented a more refined and effective open-tube endoscope. According to Nezhat, Desormeaux's pioneering contribution was the creation of the first functional endoscope and earned him the title of "father of endoscopy". Desormeaux called the process of using his device *"l'endoscopie"* (The endoscopy), coining the term for future generations. Desormeaux presented his device to the Academy of Science in Paris in 1853. The times were different now, and Desormeaux did not face the resentment and politics experienced by Bozzini.

1.3.3 Modern Laparoscopy

The twentieth century started off with Georg Kelling (1866–1945), a surgeon and gastroenterologist, giving a lecture to the Society of German Natural Scientists and Physicians in Hamburg, Germany. This was at their 73rd annual meeting in 1901 [24, 25]. After delivering his lecture "On the inspection of the gullet and the stomach with flexible instruments" [26], Kelling proceeded to demonstrate his laparoscopic technique on a dog. According to Schollmeyer et al., he referred to his procedure as "coelioscopy."

Kelling had the advantage of studying under and working with some of the leading innovators in medical research. Some of those innovations were eventually added and integrated into Kelling's process. For example, he utilized the lighting of

---

[4] Several sources spell Bozzini's first name as "Phillip," a conventional spelling. Another source used the spelling as "Phillippe" while another used Philip. However, the correct spelling appears to be Philipp. Part of the problem may be that most of the original documents are in German and translators may have used a spelling with which they were more familiar. A seemingly trivial matter, but important, when researching a specific individual.

the Max Nitze cystoscope as well as the trocar developed by Alfred Fiedler. Both these tools, plus his insufflation device were part of his introduction to the examination of the esophagus of the dog after his lecture in 1901. For these reasons, Kelling is frequently referred to as the "inventor of modern laparoscopy" giving "birth" to the field of laparoscopy. One unusual aspect of Kelling's work and research was his willingness to collaborate and exchange ideas with other scholars in the field, something rarely done [27].

Dimitri Oscarovic Ott (1855–1929) was a Russian physician and gynecologist who developed a procedure he called "ventroscopy" [28] and one of the lesser known pioneers of laparoscopic surgery. He was a contemporary of Kelling and Jacobaeus but was already putting his ideas into practice while the other two were just beginning to present their research. Ott's technique involved making a single incision in the cul-de-sac and then used a head lamp to inspect the abdominal cavity. According to Hatzinger, Ott is considered to be the father of the Russian school of OB/GYN and founder of laparoscopic and endoscopic surgery in Russia. Ott is also considered to be one of the founders of the idea of natural orifices transluminal endoscopic surgery (NOTES) [29].

While this chapter has focused primarily on the people who pioneered laparoscopic surgery, there are some important ideas as well, not specifically associated with one individual. The idea of minimally invasive surgery is well established, but now there is a push for "ultra-minimally invasive" surgery. According to Halim and Tavakkolizadeh, the idea is to use more advanced endoscopes and natural orifices to achieve "scarless" surgery. Ever since the advent of laparoscopy and endoscopy, the effort has always been minimum trauma and resulting to less pain.

Hans Christian Jacobaeus (1879–1937) was a contemporary with many of the pioneers of laparoscopy and the first to perform laparoscopic surgery in Stockholm, Sweden [30]. He is credited with coining the term "laparoscopy". He published his initial work on a dog in 1910. Jacobaeus used a Nitze cystoscope, like that used by Kelling. He was also very concerned about possible damage that could be done with a trocar, so he focused on corpses and animals. He pushed for the development of more effective laparoscopic tools. As an enthusiastic supporter of the ideas of laparoscopy, Jacobaeus became one of the best-known pioneers and experts in the field. He did, however, acknowledge the work and ideas of Kelling.

Bertram M. Bernheim (1880–1958) is considered to be one of the most influential endoscopic pioneers and contemporary with Jacobaeus. Practicing at Johns Hopkins University Hospital, he was the first American to perform laparoscopy in the U.S. in 1911. Bernheim preferred to describe what he did as "organoscopy". Bernheim first used a proctoscope, a metal tube with the end blunted, to examine the intra-abdominal area in dogs. The tool also had an electric light, but he was unhappy with its performance. Bernheim then developed his own endoscopic instrument, which he called the "organoscope" [31].

Kurt Semm (1927–2003) was born in Munich, Germany and completed his medical education at the Ludwig-Maximillian University School of Medicine in 1951 [32]. Semm's medical specialty was obstetrics and Gynecology. He built a number of instruments and one of his creations resulted in much attention. The instrument was a CO_2 electric insufflator, developed in 1956. Semm focused on the development of numerous technical innovations that would be of help in his gynecological work, as well as the development of tools and techniques to bring about "endoscopic hemostasis". According to Litynski, there was a great deal of resistance to his work, and that resistance hit a peak when Semm performed the first laparoscopic appendectomy in 1980.[5]

Antoniou et al. argued that Semm (1927–2003) transformed the use of laparoscopy by demonstrating its value as a therapeutic surgical process and not just a diagnostic tool. Antoniou et al. also argued that Semm's use of laparoscopy as a surgical tool opened the eyes of others such as Mouret and Mühe to use laparoscopy for other surgical procedures. The idea of using laparoscopy for surgery rather than just diagnosis was not always well received, and there were a few complications that aided his detractors. However, Semm continued his work and research and developed better laparoscopic equipment.

Sources referencing Semm's work all note the harassment he experienced at the hands of his peers and even his own chief of service [32, 33]. Some of the criticism may have stemmed from a few cases of bowel injury from the laparoscopy. Regardless, Semm continued his work, and his research was eventually accepted and are now widespread practice. Semm's research and presentation of his work opened the door for many others to consider laparoscopy as a surgical treatment tool. According to Himal [34], the beginning of the use of laparoscopy for cholecystectomy was one of the most significant medical events in history. Phillipe Mouret [35], a French surgeon, in discussing the development of laparoscopic cholecystectomy [36] gave credit to the development of video in helping others better understand the technical procedures. Mouret argued that endoscopic cholecystectomy was as safe as or safer than an open surgery.

Who conducted the first laparoscopic cholecystectomy seems to be a point of some controversy. For many years, Phillipe Mouret was given credit for performing the first laparoscopic cholecystectomy in 1987 [37]. In March of that year, he performed his first laparoscopic cholecystectomy on a 50-year-old woman [38]. To Mouret's surprise, when he visited the patient the next morning, she was dressed and ready to go home. This last point was the key as it was clear that laparoscopy offered the potential for less trauma and faster recovery.

---

[5]The actual date when Semm performed the laparoscopic appendectomy is not clear. Multiple sources vary. According to some, the surgery took place in 1981 when Semm performed the first laparoscopic appendectomy. Others provide a different and usually more specific date. For example, on September 13, 1980, Kurt Semm performed the world's first laparoscopic appendicectomy at the University of Kiel in Germany. Arezzo provide the date of September 12, 1980. However, in two sources, one of which Semm was ostensibly a contributor, it was stated that the procedure occurred on May 30, 1980. Several sources give the date as 1983. However, that is most likely because that was the date of the published article by Semm. However, nowhere in that article did Semm discuss the date of his presentation. The article is a description of his methodology. The likely date is September 1980.

However, in Germany, "Erich Mühe claimed the execution of the first laparoscopic cholecystectomy on September 12, 1985" [5] p. 254. Polychronidis et al. stated that the first laparoscopic cholecystectomy took place in March 1987 in Lyon, France, and Philippe Mouret was the physician. Additional sources backed the claim that Mühe was the first stating that Dr. Med Erich Mühe of Böblingen, Germany, performed the first laparoscopic cholecystectomy on September 12, 1985 [39]. One problem for Mühe was that the German Surgical Society rejected his work in 1986 after he reported that he had performed the first laparoscopic cholecystectomy, yet in 1992 he received their highest award, the German Surgical Society Anniversary Award.

In 1990, in Atlanta, at the Society of American Gastrointestinal Surgeons (SAGES) Convention, Perissat, Berci, Cuschieri, Dubois, and Mouret were all recognized by SAGES for performing early laparoscopic cholecystectomies, but Mühe was not. However, in 1999, he was recognized by SAGES for having performed the first laparoscopic cholecystectomy. SAGES invited Mühe to present the Storz Lecture. In Mühe's presentation, titled "'The First Laparoscopic Cholecystectomy,'" which he gave in March 1999 in San Antonio, Texas, he described the first procedure. Finally, Mühe had received the worldwide acclaim that he deserved for his pioneering work" [39] p. 89.

1.4 Laparoscopic Colectomy

Laparoscopic cholecystectomy has evolved to become the most common laparoscopic surgical procedure. In the United States, gallbladder removal or cholecystectomy is among the ten most common laparoscopic surgical procedures [40]. Similar is the case in the medical world of Western countries. Laparoscopic colectomy, however, has not become a preferred method of surgery yet and most of the surgeons choose the open method. The first laparoscopic colectomy was operated 5 years after the first cholecystectomy because of anatomical and physiological difficulties of the colon. In June 1990, surgeon Moises Jacobs was the first to perform laparoscopic colonic resection in Miami, Florida. It was in October of the same year that Dr. Dennis Fowler performed a laparoscopic sigmoid resection. In 1991, surgeons Jacobs, Verdeja, and Goldstein operated the first laparoscopic colectomy [41].

Although 26 years have passed since the first laparoscopic colectomy, the prevalence of this technique is still very low, and most surgeons are hesitant to perform a colectomy laparoscopically. Technological advancements have contributed to the improvement of laparoscopic colectomy technique. In the beginning, the risk of intra-operative bleeding was very high with many incidences of bowel and vascular injuries after trocar insertion or with cases of thermal injury to the bowel because of cauterization. The increase in experience and surgical skills' improvement have increased the number of colectomies surgeons perform laparoscopically. However, the general number remains low. In the United States, surgeons perform only one-third of colon resections laparoscopically despite the clinical evidence and publications about safety, efficacy, and benefits of the surgical technique [42]. Similar to the hesitation of using laparoscopy for surgery rather than just diagnosis during Semm's time in the nineteenth century, the idea of laparoscopic colectomy is still not well received. Steps need to be taken for surgeons to endorse laparoscopic colectomy as a surgical technique offering to their patients less trauma and pain and fewer days of hospitalization.

Training is critical in this type of surgery because of the complexity of the anatomy. Surgeons achieve the learning curve of laparoscopic colectomy after 30 to 36 cases [43], whereas with laparoscopic cholecystectomy surgeons reach the learning curve after 15 cases [44]. Because of the anatomical difficulties, the learning curve of the laparoscopic colectomy is stiffer, more demanding, and therefore more training is required to achieve optimal results from admission to discharge. According to the American Society of Colon and Rectal Surgeons (ASCRS) and the Society of American Gastrointestinal and Endoscopic Surgeons (SAGES), surgeons should perform 20 to 70 laparoscopic colectomies to acquire the necessary skills [45]. Nevertheless, surgeons perform on average less than 11 laparoscopic colectomies a year, a number insufficient for surgical skills' acquisition and development.

Simulators have emerged as an adjunct to the operating room training method to meet the evolving needs of contemporary health care systems like effectiveness, quality of treatment, and cost-containment. Research has indicated that training with virtual reality simulators leads in less postoperative complications and decrease of the total cost of treatment [46]. The history of laparoscopic colectomy is relatively new. However, increasing number of colon cancers and benign tumors, plus the demand for minimal invasive surgery, generates an urge for additional training in laparoscopic colectomy. This is especially true after published clinical evidence that the outcomes of the laparoscopic surgery are the same or better than those of open surgery, and open surgery causes more trauma, pain, days of hospitalization, and cost.

1.5   Conclusion

Surgery has advanced from flints and twigs to sophisticated operations because of revolutionary technologies and advanced medical instruments. The introduction of robotic surgery in colonic disease has shown similarly positive results as laparoscopic surgery [47–49]. Robotic surgery finds an increasing number of applications. In the future, computer consoles may allow surgeons to operate on a patient from far away, making telesurgery a preferred and economical method of surgery. Technological advancements outpace surgeons' knowledge and skills. Therefore, contemporary surgeons are confronted with the need to identify resources and allocate them to intensified, advanced, and continuous training that can help them acquire the necessary skills and competencies to meet the needs of their patients, who become more knowledgeable and demanding.

In this brief chapter of the history of laparoscopic surgery, the discussion was focused primarily on key individuals who made major innovative steps in facilitating the implementation of laparoscopic surgery. Some, such as Kelling, Jacobaeus, and Semm appear to have affected the entire practice of MIS. Others developed unique approaches within the context of their own country. However, it is not possible to acknowledge the contributions of the hundreds of pioneers. If interested, please review the references for this chapter and read further.

References

1. Harrell AG, Heniford BT. Minimally invasive abdominal surgery: lux et veritas past, present, and future. Am J Surg. 2005;190(2):239–43. https://doi.org/10.1016/j.amjsurg.2005.05.019.
2. Sgambati SA, Ballantyne GH. Minimally invasive surgery for diseases of the colon & rectum: the legacy of an ancient tradition. In: Jager RM, Wexner S, editors. Laparoscopic colectomy. New York, NY: Churchill & Livingstone; 1995. p. 13–23.
3. Antoniou SA, Antoniou GA, Antoniou AI, Granderath FA. Past, present, and future of minimally invasive abdominal surgery [commentary]. JSLS. 2015;19(3):1–5. https://doi.org/10.4293/JSLS.2015.00052.
4. Spaner SJ, Warnock GL. A brief history of endoscopy, laparoscopy, and laparoscopic surgery. J Laparoendosc Adv Surg Tech A. 1997;7(6):369–73. https://doi.org/10.1089/lap.1997.7.369.
5. Arezzo A. The past, the present, and the future of minimally invasive therapy in laparoscopic surgery: a review and speculative outlook. Minim Invasive Ther Allied Technol. 2014;23(5):253–60. https://doi.org/10.3109/13645706.2014.900084.
6. Antoniou SA, Antoniou GA, Koutras C, Antoniou I. Endoscopy and laparoscopy: a historical aspect of medical terminology. Surg Endosc. 2012;26(12):3650–4. https://doi.org/10.1007/s00464-012-2389-y.
7. Wikipedia. List of Greek and Latin roots in English. 2017. https://en.wikipedia.org/wiki/List_of_Greek_and_Latin_roots_in_English.
8. Nezhat C. Nezhat's history of endoscopy: a historical analysis of endoscopy's ascension since antiquity. Tuttlingen: Endo Press; 2011.
9. Channel4. History of surgery. 2013. http://www.channel4.com/explore/surgerylive/history.html.
10. Tuffs A. Kurt Semm [obituary]. Br Med J. 2003;327(7411):397–8. https://doi.org/10.1136/bmj.327.7411.397.
11. Papaziogas TV. History of surgery [Greek]. Thessaloniki, GR: University Studio Press; 1981.
12. Toledo-Pereyra LH. The soul of the knife: the essence, the being of the surgical profession. J Investig Surg. 2003;16(1):1–2. https://doi.org/10.1080/08941930390153014.
13. University of Virginia. Surgical instruments from ancient Rome. 2007. http://exhibits.hsl.virginia.edu/romansurgical/.
14. Galen. In: Green RM, Translator. A translation of Galen's hygiene: De sanitate tuenda. Springfield, IL: Charles C. Thomas; 1951.
15. Gordon AG, Magos AL. The development of laparoscopic surgery. Baillieres Clin Obstet Gynaecol. 1989;3(3):429–49.
16. Lau WY, Leow CK, Li AKC. History of endoscopic and laparoscopic surgery. World J Surg. 1997;21(4):444–53. https://doi.org/10.1007/PL00012268.
17. Nakajima K, Milson JW, Böhm B. History of laparoscopic surgery. In: Milsom JW, Böhm B, Nakajima K, editors. Laparoscopic colorectal surgery. 2nd ed. New York, NY: Springer Science+Business Media, Inc.; 2006. p. 1–9.
18. Nano M. A brief history of laparoscopy. G Chir. 2012;33(3):53–7.
19. Qari M. Abul Qasim Khalaf ibn al-Abbas al- Zahrawi (Abulcasis). J Appl Hematol. 2010;1(1):66–7.
20. Nezhad GSM, Dalfardi B, Ghanizadeh A, Golzari SEJ. Insights into Avicenna's knowledge of gastrointestinal medicine and his account of an enema device. Acta Med Hist Adriat. 2015;13(Supl. 2):29–40.
21. Morgenstern L. The 200th anniversary of the first endoscope: Philipp Bozzini (1773–1809). Surg Innov. 2005a;12(2):105–6. https://doi.org/10.1177/155335060501200201.

22. Cengiz F. Same surgery - altered techniques; past, present and future of laparoscopic and endoscopic surgery. J Clin Anal Med. 2013;4(1):72–5.
23. Modlin IM, Kidd M, Lye KD. From the lumen to the laparoscope. Arch Surg. 2004;139(10):1110–26. https://doi.org/10.1001/archsurg.139.10.1110.
24. Hatzinger M, Badawi JK, Häcker A, Langbein S, Honeck P, Alken P. Georg Kelling (1866-1945): the inventor of modern laparoscopy [German]. Urologe. 2006;45(7):868–71. https://doi.org/10.1007/s00120-006-1068-9.
25. Schollmeyer T, Soyinka AS, Schollmeyer M, Meinhold-Heerlein I. Georg Kelling (1866–1945): the root of modern day minimal invasive surgery. A forgotten legend? Arch Gynecol Obstet. 2007;276(5):505–9. https://doi.org/10.1007/s00404-007-0372-y.
26. Kelling G. Endoscopy of the oesophagus and stomach. Lancet. 1900;155(4000):1189–98. https://doi.org/10.1016/S0140-6736(01)96860-6.
27. Litynski GS. Kurt Semm and the fight against skepticism: endoscopic hemostasis, laparoscopic appendectomy, and Semm's impact on the "laparoscopic revolution". JSLS. 1998;2(3):309–13.
28. Hatzinger M, Fesenko A, Büger L, Sohn M. Dimitrij Oscarovic Ott (1855–1929) "Ventroscopy": his contribution to development of laparoscopy [German]. Urologe. 2013;52(10):1454–8. https://doi.org/10.1007/s00120-013-3224-3.
29. Halim I, Tavakkolizadeh A. NOTES: the next surgical revolution? Int J Surg. 2008;6(4):273–2796. https://doi.org/10.1016/j.ijsu.2007.10.002.
30. Hatzinger M, Häcker A, Langbein S, Kwon S, Hoang-Böhm J, Alken P. Hans-Christian Jacobaeus (1879-1937): the inventor of human laparoscopy and thoracoscopy [German]. Urologe. 2006;45(9):1184–6. https://doi.org/10.1007/s00120-006-1069-8.
31. Morgenstern L. The first laparoscopist in the United States: Bertram M. Bernheim, MD. Surg Innov. 2007;14(4):241–2. https://doi.org/10.1177/1553350607309433.
32. Bhattacharya K. Kurt Semm: a laparoscopic crusader. J Minim Access Surg. 2007;3(1):35–6. https://doi.org/10.4103/0972-9941.30686.
33. Kavic MS, Kavic SM, Kavic SM. Laparoscopic appendectomy. In: Wettner PA, editor. Prevention & management of laparoendoscopic surgical complications [iBook]. 3rd ed; 2010. http://laparoscopy.blogs.com/prevention_management_3/2010/08/laparoscopic-appendectomy.html.
34. Himal HS. Minimally invasive (laparoscopic) surgery. Surg Endosc. 2002;16(12):1647–52. https://doi.org/10.1007/s00464-001-8275-7.
35. Mouret P. From the first laparoscopic cholecystectomy to the frontiers of laparoscopic surgery: the future prospectives. Dig Surg. 1991;8(2):124–5. https://doi.org/10.1159/000172015.
36. Mouret P. How I developed laparoscopic cholecystectomy. Annu Acad Med. 1996;25(5):744–7.
37. Blum CA, Adams DB. Who did the first laparoscopic cholecystectomy? J Minim Access Surg. 2011;7(3):165–8. https://doi.org/10.4103/0972-9941.83506.
38. Reynolds W Jr. The first laparoscopic cholecystectomy. JSLS. 2001;5(1):89–94.
39. Health Grades. The most common surgeries in the U. S, 2016. www.healthgrades.com/explore/the-10-most-common-surgeris-in-the-us.
40. Jacobs M, Verdeja JC, Goldstein HS. Minimally invasive colon resection (laparoscopic colectomy). Surg Laparosc Endosc Percutan Tech. 1991;1(3):144–50.
41. Pedraza R, Nieto J, Malave V, Haas EM. The current status of laparoscopic versus open colectomy: Incidence and short-term outcomes in a cohort of 59,000 patients. Poster presented at SAGES with program number P122. 2014. https://www.sages.org/meetings/annual-meeting/abstracts-archive/the-current-status-of-laparoscopic-versus-open-colectomy-incidence-and-short-term-outcomes-in-a-cohort-of-59000-patients/.
42. Haas EM, Nieto J, Ragupath M, Aminian A, Patel CB. Critical appraisal of learning curve for single incision laparoscopic right colectomy. Surg Endosc. 2013;27(12):4499–503. https://doi.org/10.1007/s00464-013-3096-z.
43. Deutsch GB, Sathyanarayana SA, Giangola M, Akerman M, DeNoto G III, Klein JDS, Rubach E. Competence acquisition for single-incision laparoscopic cholecystectomy. JSLS. 2015;19(1):e2014–6. https://doi.org/10.4293/JSLS.2014.00116.

44. Pendlimari R, Holubar SD, Dozois EJ, Larson DW, Pemberton JH, Cima RR. Technical proficiency in hand-assisted laparoscopic colon and rectal surgery: determining how many cases are required to achieve mastery. Arch Surg. 2012;147(4):317–22. https://doi.org/10.1001/archsurg.2011.879.
45. Matsiota EJ. Laparoscopic colectomy training: a quasi-experimental comparison of simulators to traditional training. 2015. http://search.proquest.com/docview/1706722295?accountid=35812.
46. Brody F, Richards NG. Review of robotic versus conventional laparoscopic surgery. Surg Endosc. 2014;28(5):1413–24. https://doi.org/10.1007/s00464-013-3342-4.
47. Deutsch GB, Sathyanarayana SA, Gunabushanam V, Mishra N, Rubach E, Zemon H, et al. Robotic vs. laparoscopic colorectal surgery: an institutional experience. Surg Endosc. 2012;26(4):956–63. https://doi.org/10.1007/s00464-011-1977-6.
48. Zarak A, Castillo A, Kichler K, de la Cruz L, Tamariz L, Kaza S. Robotic versus laparoscopic surgery for colonic disease: a meta-analysis of postoperative variables. Surg Endosc. 2015;29(6):1341–7. https://doi.org/10.1007/s00464-015-4197-7.
49. Smith GE. The most ancient splints. Br Med J. 1908;1(2465):732–4, 736-731, 736-732.

Types of Colon Surgery and Anatomy

Dimitrios Mantas, Ioannis D. Kostakis, and Zoi Garoufalia

2.1 Introduction

Laparoscopic colectomy both for benign and malignant diseases, located in any part of the colon, has gained popularity over the past years. Comparing with the open surgical procedures, there are no differences concerning the anatomical point of view, in order to achieve similar oncologic results. Nevertheless, there are different approaches based on surgeon's experience to regain the most of the laparoscopic advantages, as well as differentiations in patients' and surgeons' position during every specific operation. Even though the main goal is the same comparing open and laparoscopic procedures, the last provide better visualization with minor surgical trauma, especially for difficult anatomical sites. It is well known among surgeons that colorectal cancer remains the third most common cancer and the third most common cause of cancer-related mortality worldwide [1]. On the other hand, there are several benign disorders that necessitate colectomy for cure. The implementation of laparoscopic surgery as compared to open procedures has the benefit of minimal trauma, reduced recovery time, and less wound complications. There is no time benefit when comparing the two methods as well as the oncological results [2]. However, the laparoscopic method has the drawback of the longer operative time. The treatment of benign disease of the colon with laparoscopic colectomy is widely accepted. Colon cancer can be adequately treated laparoscopically as long as the oncologic principles are not violated. The average mortality, following laparoscopic colorectal surgery, is less than 2%. Lacy et al. in a randomized trial reported that perioperative mortality was 1% for laparoscopic resection and 3% for open

D. Mantas (✉) · I. D. Kostakis · Z. Garoufalia
Faculty of Medicine, 2nd Propedeutic Surgical Department, Laiko General Hospital, National and Kapodistrian University of Athens, Athens, Greece
e-mail: dvmantas@med.uoa.gr

© The Editor(s) (if applicable) and The Author(s),
under exclusive license to Springer Nature Switzerland AG 2021
G. Kouraklis, E. (J.) Matsiota (eds.), *Laparoscopic Colon Surgery*,
https://doi.org/10.1007/978-3-030-56728-6_2

resection [3]. The Clinical Outcome of Surgical Therapy (COST) trial, a multiinstitutional study, proved that when colon cancer was the issue, laparoscopic colectomy and open colectomy had the same recurrent rates which suggest that laparoscopic surgery compared to open surgery is an acceptable choice [4]. Furthermore, laparoscopic colectomy has the benefit of less hospital stay and postoperative pain, resulting in an earlier return to regular activity (sooner rehabilitation). Regarding pulmonary function there is faster recovery and lower incidence of surgical site complications.

The types of laparoscopic colectomy depend mainly in the site of the tumor taking into consideration the main vascular supply in order to have the best oncological result.

2.2   Anatomy of Colon and Rectum

The large intestine extends from the terminal ileum to the anus (Fig. 2.1). Its length reaches 1.5 m and comprises the following segments: cecum, colon (ascending, transverse, descending, and sigmoid), and rectum. The segment of the large intestine below the ileocecal valve is the cecum. It is approximately 5 cm in length with a 7.5 cm in its greater diameter and lies in the right lower quadrant of the abdomen. The segment of the large intestine above the ileocecal valve is the ascending colon, which lies in the right abdominal flank. Peritoneum covers only its anterior surface and it is fused to the abdominal wall posteriorly. The next segment, the transverse colon, extends from the hepatic flexure, which is located beneath the right hepatic lobe and anteriorly to the duodenum, to the splenic flexure, which is located near the

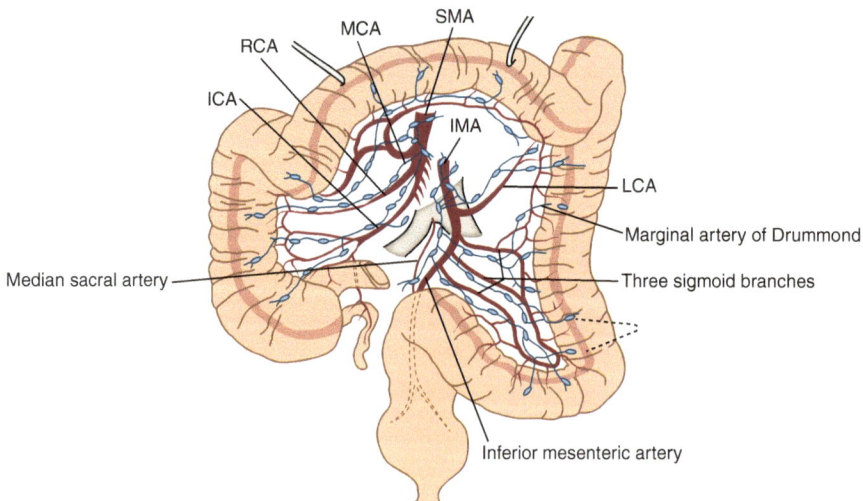

Fig. 2.1 Colon segments and vessels [5]

posterolateral surface of the spleen and the pancreatic tail and is attached to the left hemidiaphragm with the phrenicocolic ligament. The transverse colon, lies in front of the pancreas, is connected with the greater gastric curvature through the gastro-colic ligament, which is part of the greater omentum and has a mesentery that reaches the posterior wall of the lesser sac. The descending colon lies in the left abdominal flank. Peritoneum covers its anterior and lateral surfaces and it is fused to the abdominal wall posteriorly. The left iliac crest marks the transitions of the descending colon to the sigmoid colon. The sigmoid colon lies in the left lower quadrant of the abdomen. It has a mesentery and the left ureter crosses its base. The next and final segment of the large intestine is the rectum, which is located inside the pelvis and also has its own mesentery. It is about 12 cm long and begins at the retrosigmoid junction, which is located in front of the third sacral vertebra accord-ing to the anatomists and at the level of the sacral promontory according to the surgeons and ends at the puborectalis sling, where the anus begins. The ureters are close to the rectum at the pelvic inlet. Peritoneum covers the upper third of the rec-tum, whereas the lower two-thirds are extraperitoneal. The parietal peritoneum forms the *pouch of Douglas* or *cul-de-sac* as it passes from the ventral surface of the rectum to the dorsal surface of the uterus in females and the bladder and the seminal vesicles in males [6–8] (Fig. 2.1).

2.2.1 Vascular System of the Colon Arterial Supply

The superior mesenteric artery supplies blood to the cecum, the ascending colon, and the transverse colon, whereas the inferior mesenteric artery supplies blood to the descending colon, the sigmoid colon, and a large part of rectum. The boundary between the two arterial supplies is the splenic flexure. Specifically, the ileocolic and the right colic artery, which arise from the superior mesenteric artery, supply the cecum and the ascending colon. The middle colic artery, which arises from the superior mesenteric artery, supplies the transverse colon. The distal part of the trans-verse colon and the splenic flexure receive blood from the middle colic artery in one-third of the cases, whereas they receive blood by the left colic artery, which arises from the inferior mesenteric artery, in two-thirds of the cases. The descending colon is supplied by the left colic artery and the sigmoid colon by the sigmoid arter-ies, which are branches of the inferior mesenteric artery. The branches of all the aforementioned arteries form anastomotic arcades that give rise to the marginal artery of Drummond, which lies in the mesocolon, close to the bowel. The rectum receives blood from the superior hemorrhoidal artery, which is the continuation of the inferior mesenteric artery, the right and left middle hemorrhoidal artery, which are branches of the right and left internal iliac artery, respectively, the right and left inferior hemorrhoidal artery, which are branches of the right and left internal puden-dal artery, respectively, and the medial sacral artery, which originates from the abdominal aorta, just above its bifurcation [6–8] (Figs. 2.1 and 2.2).

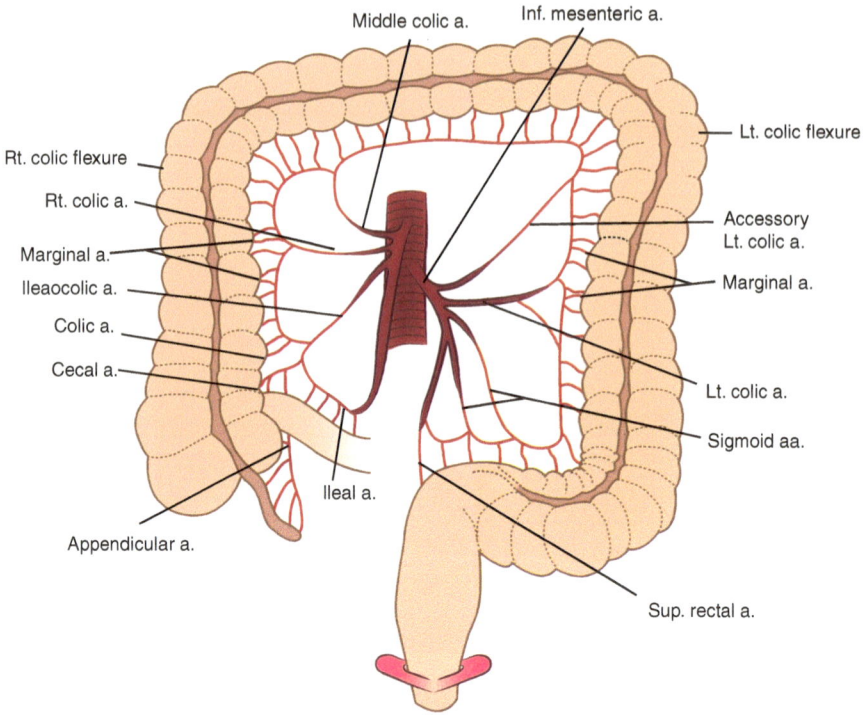

Fig. 2.2 Blood supply to the colon [7]

2.2.1.1 Venous Drainage

The distribution of the veins of the large intestine resembles that of its arteries. Thus, the ileocolic and the right colic vein receive blood from the cecum and the ascending colon, and the middle colic vein receives blood from the transverse colon. All these veins are tributaries of the superior mesenteric vein. On the other hand, the descending colon is drained by the left colic vein and the sigmoid colon is drained by the sigmoid veins. These veins are tributaries of the inferior mesenteric vein. The blood returning from the rectum is collected by the superior hemorrhoidal vein, which is the beginning of the inferior mesenteric artery, the middle hemorrhoidal veins, and the inferior hemorrhoidal veins, which form a plexus that serves as a potential portosystemic shunt [6–8].

2.2.1.2 Lymphatic Drainage

There are four stations of lymph nodes that drain the colon. These are the epicolic lymph nodes, which are under the colonic serosa, the paracolic lymph nodes, which are located along the marginal artery, the intermediate lymph nodes, which are located along the main arteries, and the principal lymph nodes, which are at the root of the superior and the inferior mesenteric artery. The rectum is drained through the posterior rectal nodes and from them to the lymph nodes of the superior hemorrhoidal artery and afterwards to the pelvic lymph nodes. There is also some drainage towards the lymph nodes of the middle and the inferior hemorrhoidal arteries. The lymphatic drainage inferiorly to the dentate line is towards the inguinal lymph nodes [6–8] (Figs. 2.1 and 2.3).

As we already mentioned above, the location of the tumor along with the main vascular supply, determine the type of colectomy to be performed. Tumor located in the right colon (cecum, ascending colon, hepatic flexure) and transverse colon should be removed with a right colectomy (Fig. 2.4a–c), tumor of the left colon (splenic flexure, descending colon, and/or sigmoid) with a left colectomy, tumor of sigmoid colon with a sigmoidectomy (Fig. 2.4d–f), while tumors of the rectum should be removed either with low anterior or abdominoperitoneal resection according to the exact site of origin.

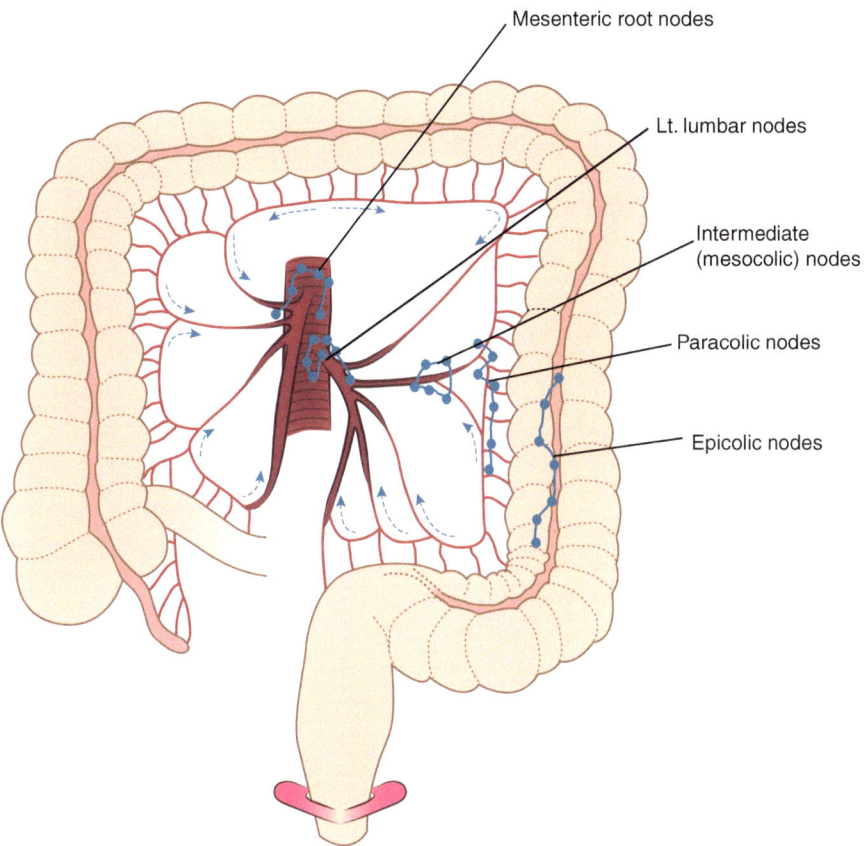

Mesenteric root nodes

Lt. lumbar nodes

Intermediate
(mesocolic) nodes

Paracolic nodes

Epicolic nodes

Fig. 2.3 The lymphatics of the colon [7]

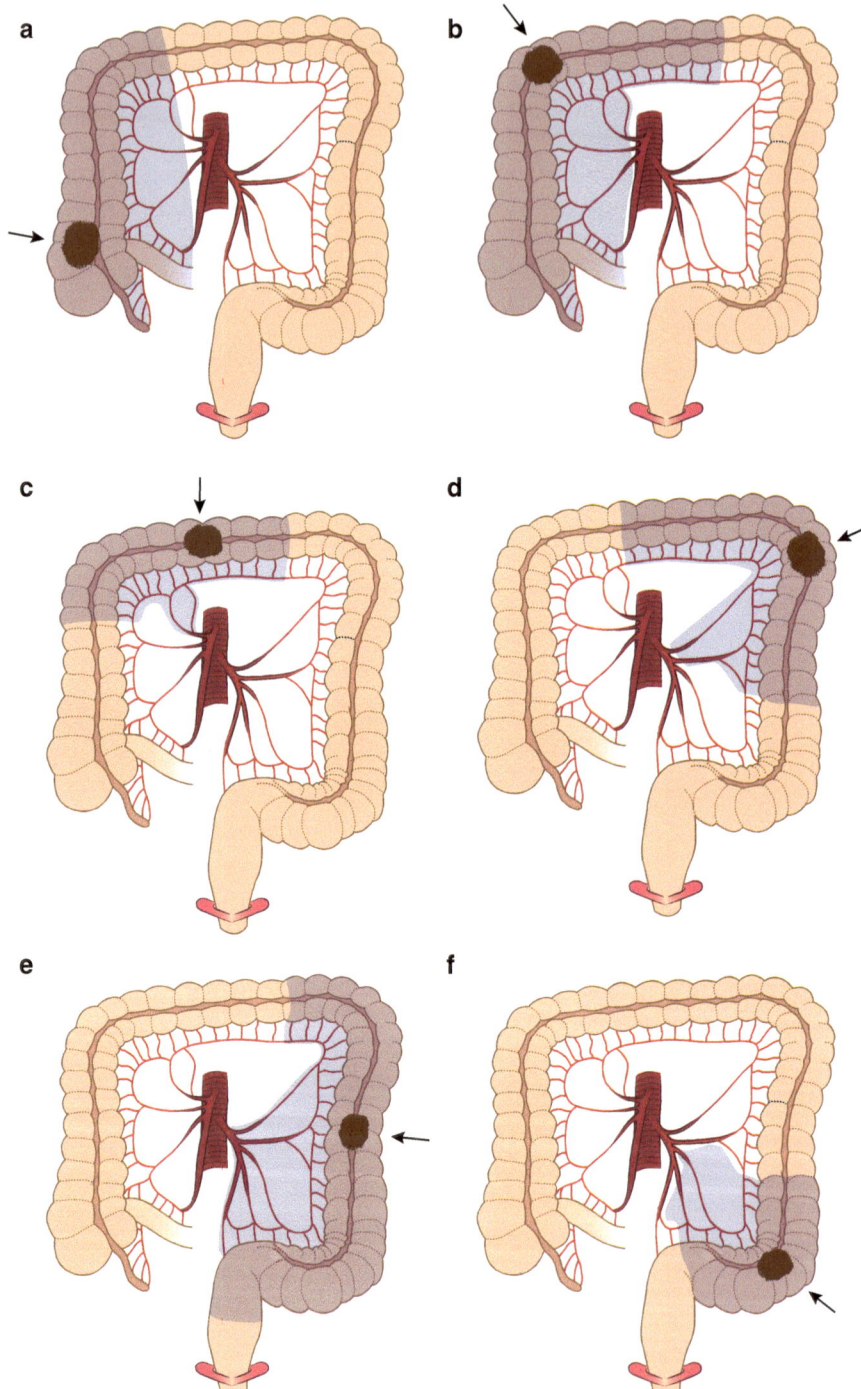

Fig. 2.4 Resection of the colon in various segments according to tumor location and major vascular supply (**a–f**) [7]

2.3   Laparoscopic Right Hemicolectomy

The patient lies in a modified lithotomy position with the lower extremities in abduction, and a nasogastric catheter and a urinary catheter are inserted [9]. The patient should be shaved and cleaned from the nipples to the pubis. The surgeon stands at the patient's left initially and between his/her legs at a later stage of the operation, whereas the opposite stands for the first assistant. The second assistant stands at the patient's left [9–11].

2.3.1   Trocar Placement

Three to five ports are placed in the following places:

- A 10 mm or 12 mm trocar above or below the umbilicus with the use of the *Veress needle*, the *Hasson technique*, or a trocar with optical obturator.
- A 5 mm trocar in the suprapubic area.
- A 10 mm or 12 mm trocar lateral to the edge of the left rectus muscle in the left lower quadrant of the abdomen.
- A fourth and even a fifth 5 mm trocar in the right lower quadrant of the abdomen (lateral to the edge of the right rectus muscle) and lateral to the margin of the left rectus muscle (4 fingerbreadths laterally to the umbilicus) [9–13].

2.3.2   Mobilization of the Cecum, Ascending Colon, and Transverse Colon

The dissection begins with the mobilization of the right colon and the transverse colon followed by the vessel ligation (lateral to medial approach) [9–11, 14–18] or may follow the opposite process (medial to lateral approach) [9–11, 13–23]. At first, the patient lies in the supine position with the head lower than the feet (Trendelenburg position). The abdomen is then examined for possible metastatic lesions, adhesions, or other pathological signs. The surgeon must also examine the small bowel with gentle maneuvers. If there are any adhesions, they are carefully divided (Fig. 2.5) [9–11, 19, 22].

Subsequently, the patient lies in the supine position with the head higher than the feet (reversed Trendelenburg position) and the left side lower than the right side. The cecum is then mobilized by grasping the terminal ileum and carefully dividing the peritoneum at the line of Toldt. The right ureter is identified and saved (Fig. 2.6).

One can use harmonic scalpel (ultrasonic shears) or electrocautery. Through gentle medial traction of the right colon, the avascular planes between the colon and the Gerota fascia (Fig. 2.7) become apparent, and the colon can be safely mobilized up to the right colic flexure (Fig. 2.8).

As the right colic flexure is mobilized, the underlying duodenum should be protected (Fig. 2.9) [9–11, 13, 17, 20–22]. Attention should also be paid to the Henle's

Fig. 2.5 Adheolysis

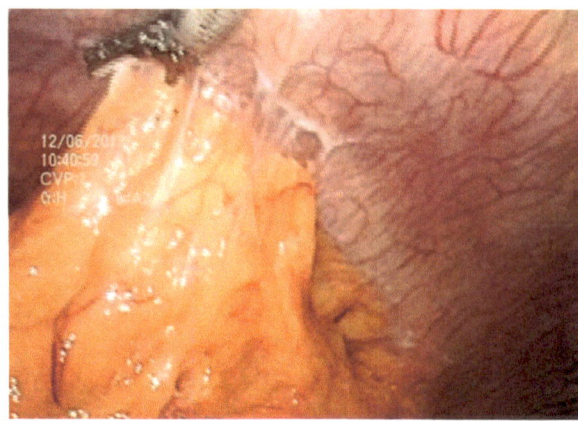

Fig. 2.6 Right ureter visualization during cecum mobilization

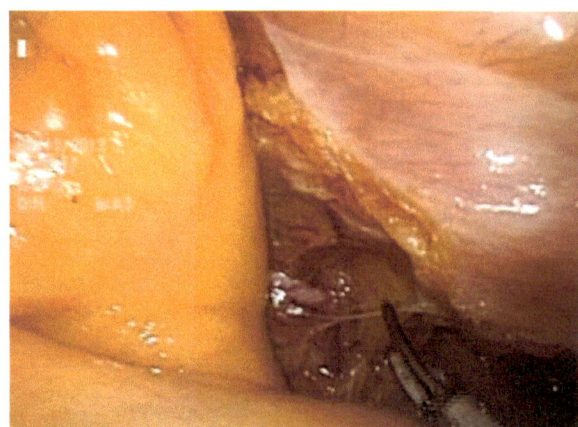

Fig. 2.7 The avascular plane between the colon and the Gerota fascia

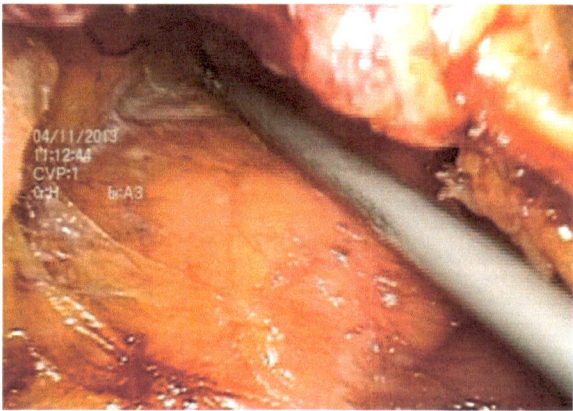

Fig. 2.8 Mobilization of
the ascending colon

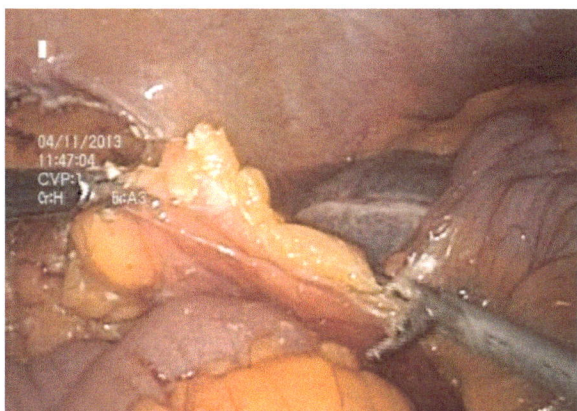

Fig. 2.9 The underlying
duodenum exposed during
colon mobilization

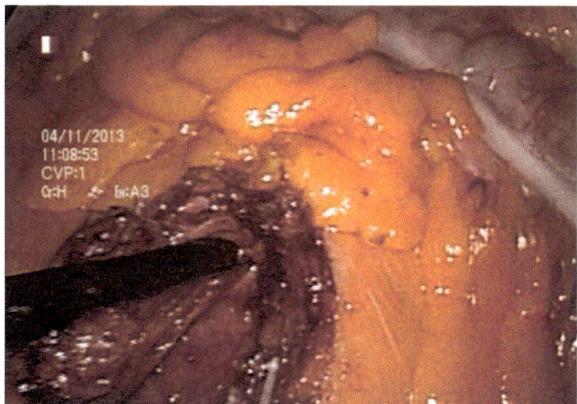

trunk, which is a vein connecting the right or middle colic vein with the right gas-
troepiploic vein [14, 17, 23]. After the right colon has been mobilized, the patient
lies in the reverse Trendelenburg position. The gastrocolic ligament is held under
tension, and the stomach is retracted anteriorly to facilitate the entrance to the lesser
sac. After the division of the gastrocolic ligament across the transverse colon, the
lesser sac is opened (Fig. 2.10). The exact site of the tumor determines the extent of
the transverse colon mobilization [9–11, 14, 18, 19, 23].

2.3.3   Vascular Approach

For vascular approach, the right colon is retracted laterally and the transverse colon
cephalad, in order for the ileocolic, right colic, and middle colic vessels to be visualized. The dissection of the ileocolic, right colic, middle colic arteries, and veins
proceeds up to their root at the superior mesenteric artery and vein, respectively.
The origin of the right colic vessels is commonly identified below the third portion

Fig. 2.10 Dissection of the gastrocolic ligament

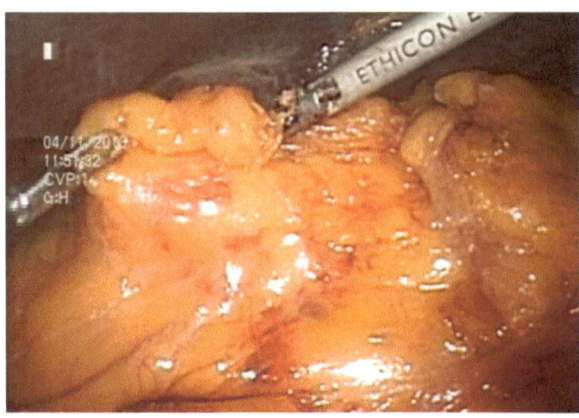

Fig. 2.11 Right colon vessels dissection

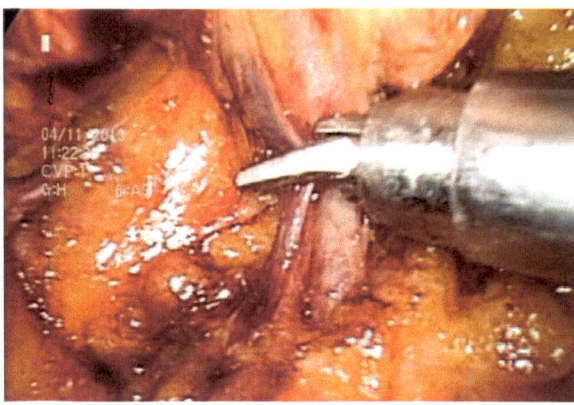

of the duodenum, and the origin of the ileocolic vessels is even lower, whereas the root of the middle colic vessels is identified above the third portion of the duodenum. The mesocolic dissection begins from the origin of the ileocolic and right colic pedicle and proceeds along the superior mesenteric vessels. The surgeon ligates the ileocolic and right colic vessels and divides 1–2 cm distal to their root using either clips and scissors or linear staplers (Fig. 2.11). Subsequently, the middle colic vessels are dissected up to their root and their right branches are ligated and divided in the same manner [9–23]. At this time, special consideration should be taken regarding variations in arterial supply (Fig. 2.12a, b).

2.3.4   Specimen Extraction, Anastomosis, and End of Operation

It is essential for the establishment of a successful ileocolic anastomosis to return the colon to its anatomic position. The patient now lies in a supine neutral position. The mobilized part of the colon is withdrawn via the umbilical port using a wound protector. The incision of the umbilical port site is extended 4–6 cm in length or a

Fig. 2.12 (**a**) Variations of the arteries to the right colon. a. usual pattern [7]. (**b**) The marginal artery is incomplete [7]

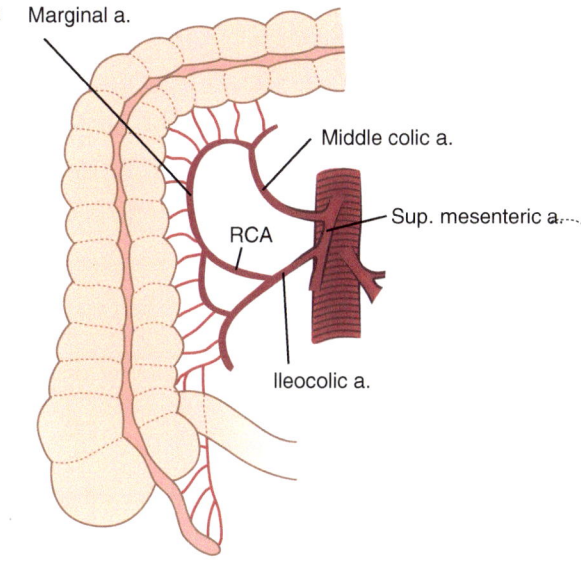

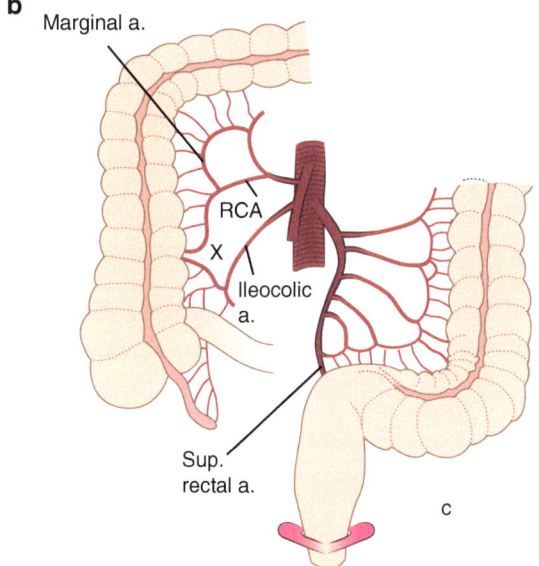

Pfannenstiel incision is performed. The distal ileum and the transverse colon are divided with a linear cutting stapler, and the specimen is extracted [9–13, 15–18, 20–23].

A tension-free, well-vascularized, side-to-side ileocolic anastomosis is then created either by a hand-sewn method or a linear stapler method. (Fig. 2.13) In the first method, an enterotomy is created in each side and their posterior and anterior edges

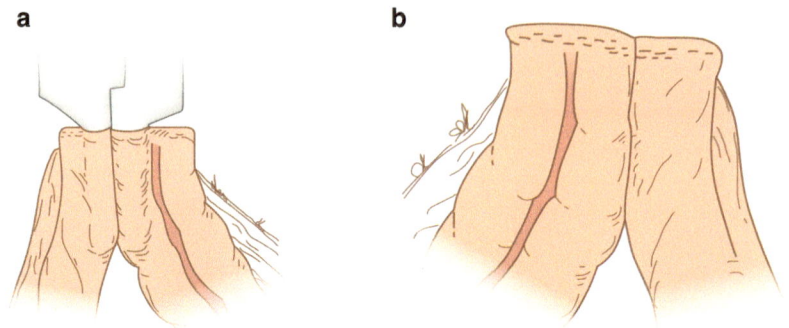

Fig. 2.13 Ileocolic anastomosis. (**a**) Alignment of colon and ileum, (**b**) Insertion of linear stapler [7]

are sutured together with running sutures, creating an anastomosis. In the second method, a small enterotomy is created in each side, through which another linear cutting stapler is inserted and creates the anastomosis, which is closed using a linear noncutting stapler outside. Twisting of the bowel and its mesentery should be avoided. Interrupted sutures are used to close the defect of the mesentery, in order to prevent internal hernia. The anastomotic site is put back to the peritoneal cavity, and the incision is closed in layers to reestablish the pneumoperitoneum. The aforementioned technique refers to extracorporeal anastomosis [9–12, 14–17, 19, 21, 22].

Alternatively, an intracorporeal anastomosis can be performed. The distal ileum and the transverse colon are divided with a laparoscopic linear cutting stapler, which is inserted through a 12 mm trocar at the left abdominal wall, and the specimen is placed in a plastic retrieval bag. The stamps of ileum and transverse colon are put together side by side by seromuscular sutures, and an enterotomy and a colotomy are made. A laparoscopic linear cutting stapler is passed through these openings and a side-to-side anastomosis is formed. The enterocolostomy is closed with interrupted or running sutures. The incision of the umbilical port site is extended 4–6 cm in length or a Pfannenstiel incision is performed and the plastic retrieval bag containing the specimen is removed. Subsequently, the incision is closed in layers to reestablish the pneumoperitoneum [12, 15–18, 20–22].

The peritoneal cavity is irrigated, and a drain may be placed in the site of the former right lateral paracolic gutter, but it is not used to be placed. The cannula sites are checked for bleeding, and the pneumoperitoneum and the cannulas are removed. The wounds are closed [9–12, 18, 22].

2.4 Laparoscopic Left Hemicolectomy and Sigmoidectomy

A modified lithotomy position is usually preferred with abduction of the patient's legs and a slight flexion of the knees. Compression stockings are used in order to prevent deep vein thrombosis. Patient's left arm is placed at an angle of 90° and the right arm is either placed at an angle of 90° or alongside the body. Paddings are used to protect the patient from nerve compression on bone prominences. The patient should be prepared from the nipples to the pubis, and a nasogastric tube and a urinary catheter are inserted. Both the primary surgeon and the second assistant stand at the patient's right side. The first assistant takes position between the patient's legs [9–11, 24–27].

2.4.1 Trocar Placement (Fig. 2.14)

Four to six trocars are inserted through the abdominal wall for laparoscopic left hemicolectomies or laparoscopic sigmoidectomies. Usually, five trocars, two with 12 mm cannula and three with 5 mm cannula are used. The first 12 mm trocar is inserted in the midline, 2–3 cm above the umbilicus, using a closed technique with the Veress needle through a 1.5–2 cm skin incision or an open technique with the Hasson method through a 1.5–2 cm skin incision and cutting through the linea alba and the parietal peritoneum or a trocar with optical obturator through a 1.5 cm skin incision. The rest trocars are inserted after the abdominal cavity is inflated with CO_2 gas and pneumoperitoneum is created. A 12 mm trocar is placed at the right lower

Fig. 2.14 Trocar placement for left colectomy [7]

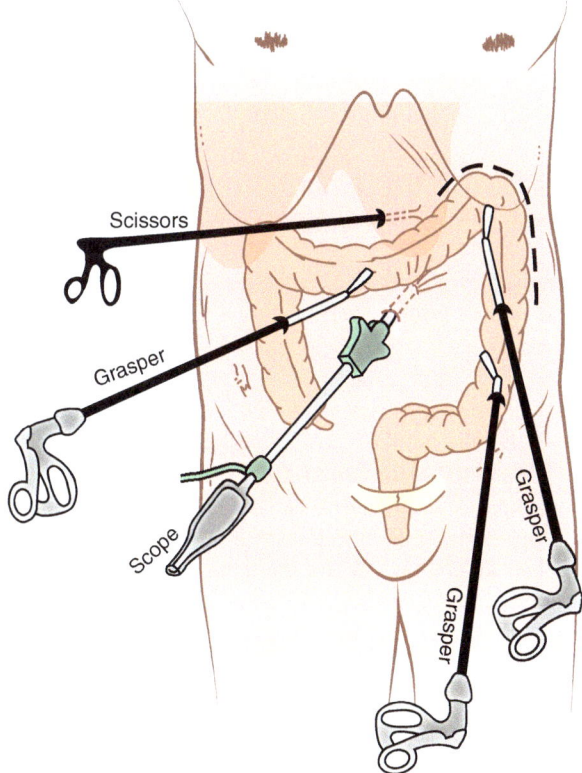

quadrant of the abdomen at the midclavicular line. Three other 5 mm trocars are inserted above the pubic symphysis, at the right of the umbilicus at the midclavicular line and at the left of the umbilicus at the midclavicular line. Alternatively, the trocar at the right of the umbilicus may be put a little higher, at the right upper quadrant at the midclavicular line, and the trocar at the left of the umbilicus may be put a little lower, at the left lower quadrant of the abdomen at the midclavicular line [9–11, 24–31].

2.4.2   Exposure of the Operative Field

The patient lies in the Trendelenburg position. This helps the placement of the small bowel, large bowel, and the greater omentum away from the operative field by using gravity. The proximal small bowel is placed in the right upper quadrant, the distal small bowel in the right lower quadrant, and the transverse colon along with the greater omentum in the left upper quadrant. These maneuvers allow the visualization of the lower abdominal aorta, the common iliac arteries, and the sacral promontory. If it is a female patient, the uterus prevents adequate exposure of the pelvis, the surgeon suspends it from the abdominal wall with sutures, either through its fundus in postmenopausal women or around the round ligaments in premenopausal women [9–11, 24–27, 29]. The dissection begins by either the dissection of the inferior mesenteric vessels and continuous with the mobilization of colon (medial to lateral approach) [9–11, 14, 19, 24–29, 32] or the opposite process, namely the mobilization of colon followed by the dissection of the inferior mesenteric vessels (lateral to medial approach) [9–11, 24–27].

2.4.3   Vascular Approach

The sigmoid mesocolon is retracted anteriorly. Thus, its base is exposed and the incision of visceral peritoneum is facilitated, which is performed from the sacral promontory up to the ligament of Treitz, along the anterior surface of the aorta. The root of the inferior mesenteric artery is exposed during this incision through dissection of the adipose tissue around it and division of the sigmoid branches of the right sympathetic trunk (Figs. 2.15 and 2.16).

The first 2–3 cm of the inferior mesenteric artery from its origin is dissected free of adipose tissue, and the artery is skeletonized, taking care not to injure the left sympathetic trunk, which is located at the left side of the artery, during this process. Subsequently, the inferior mesenteric artery is divided either at 1–2 cm distal to its root or just distal to the origin of the left colic artery. Either clips and scissors or linear staplers can be used for the division of the inferior mesenteric artery. Afterwards, the inferior mesenteric vein is recognized at the left side of the inferior mesenteric artery or at the level of the ligament of Treitz, below the pancreas. The inferior mesenteric vein is divided either proximal to the origin of the left colic vein (Fig. 2.17) or below and either clips and scissors or linear stapler can be used for its division [9–11, 14, 24–27, 29].

Fig. 2.15 Inferior mesenteric artery

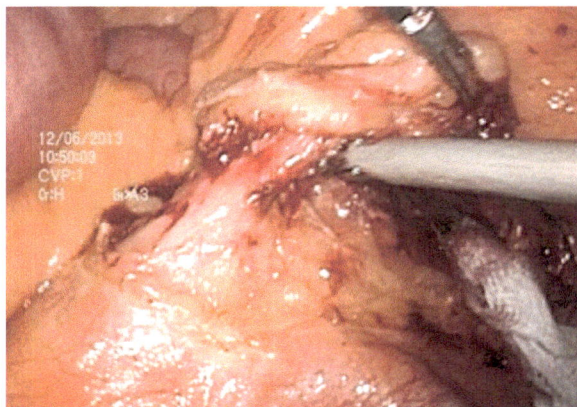

Fig. 2.16 Sigmoid vascular branches

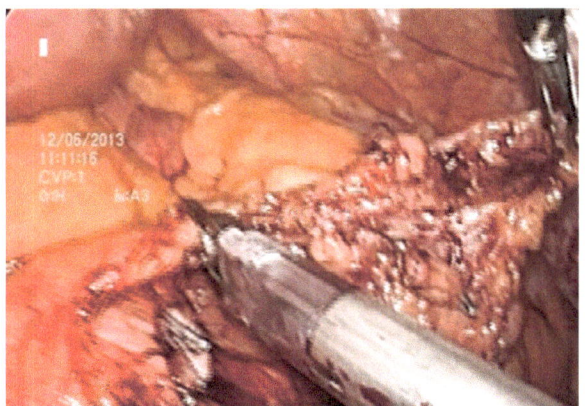

Fig. 2.17 Inferior mesenteric vein

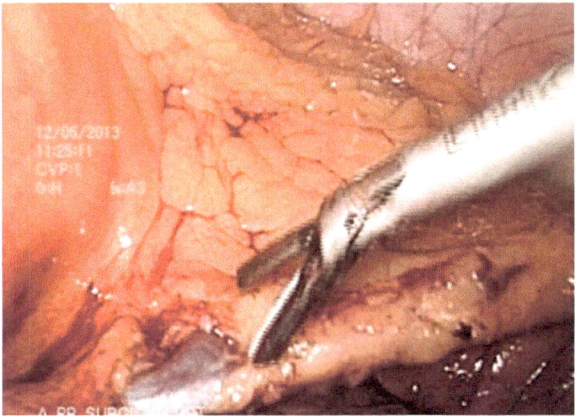

2.4.4 Mobilization of the Sigmoid and Descending Colon

After the inferior mesenteric vessels are divided, the mobilization of the sigmoid and descending colon follows by dividing its attachments posteriorly and laterally (Fig. 2.18).

The sigmoid and descending mesocolon is pulled anteriorly. The posterior space is exposed and the avascular plane between the sigmoid and descending mesocolon and Toldt's fascia is identified and divided. The dissection proceeds behind the mesocolon with a left lateral direction, towards Toldt's fascia. After the posterior mobilization, the sigmoid and descending colon is pulled to the right (Figs. 2.19 and 2.20).

This maneuver exposes Toldt's fascia, along which the dissection proceeds, cephalad and caudally until it reaches the plane of the previous medial dissection. During this mobilization, the left ureter and the left gonadal vessels should be protected [9–11, 24–27, 29].

Fig. 2.18 Mobilization of the descending colon

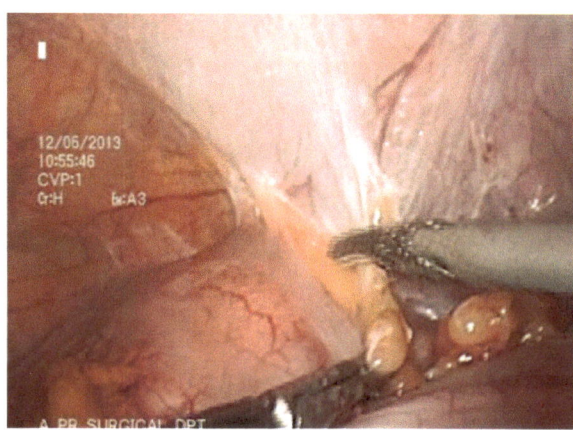

Fig. 2.19 Proximal descending colon dissection

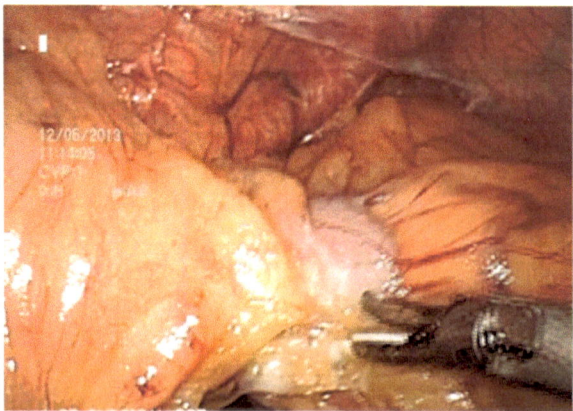

Fig. 2.20 Mobilization of the sigmoid colon

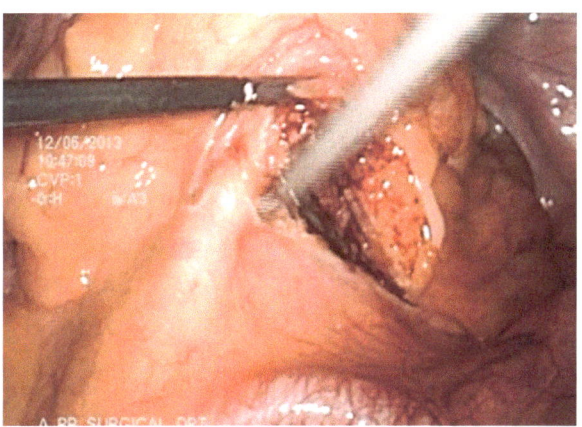

2.4.5 Mobilization of the Splenic Flexure

When a long segment of the sigmoid colon or the descending colon is resected, mobilization of the splenic flexure is necessary. This is performed through a medial or a lateral approach and by placing the patient in the reversed Trendelenburg tilt. The lateral approach begins with the transection of the lateral attachments of the descending colon. The splenic flexure and the descending colon are retracted towards the right iliac fossa and Toldt's fascia, the phrenicocolic ligament, and the gastrocolic ligament are divided. The dissection of the posterior attachments of the distal transverse and the descending colon follows next. On the other hand, the medial approach begins with the dissection of the posterior attachments of the descending and the distal transverse colon, which follows cephalad the plane created during the preceding mobilization of the sigmoid and descending colon. Retraction of the transverse colon anteriorly follows next and the inferior border of the pancreas is identified, above which the transverse mesocolon is transected and the lesser sac is opened. Subsequently, the posterior attachments of the distal transverse colon and descending colon are divided. After these maneuvers, the aforementioned lateral mobilization follows [9–11, 14, 24–27, 29].

2.4.6 Dissection of the Upper Mesorectum and Resection of the Specimen

For the dissection of the upper mesorectum, the patient lies in the Trendelenburg tilt. The upper rectum is mobilized firstly by following caudally the avascular plane between the sigmoid mesocolon and the Toldt's fascia towards the posterior portion of the upper mesorectum, and then by taking down the lateral attachments of the upper rectum. During this mobilization, ureters should be protected, especially the left one, and the superior hypogastric nerves during the process [9–11, 19, 24–27, 29].

Fig. 2.21 Transection of
the upper rectum

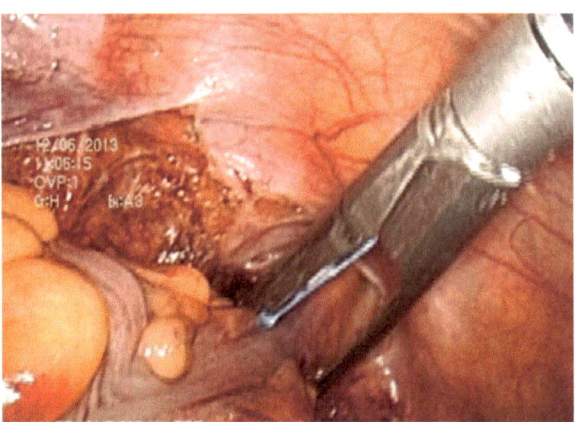

The colon is divided proximally at 10 cm or more from the tumor at the descending colon or the distal transverse colon. The mesocolon around the site of the division is transected first and then the colon. The colon is transected at an angle of 90° by using a laparoscopic linear stapler, which is inserted in the abdomen through the 12 mm trocar in the right iliac fossa. The upper rectum is divided distally at 5 cm or more from the tumor. The mesorectum around the site of division is transected first and the then the upper rectum. The upper rectum is transected at an angle of 90° by using an articulated stapler, which is inserted in the abdomen through the 12 mm trocar in the right iliac fossa (Fig. 2.21). The specimen is put in a plastic retrieval bag [9–11, 24–29, 31].

2.4.7   Extraction of the Specimen, Anastomosis, and End of Operation

The plastic retrieval bag containing the specimen is removed through a suprapubic incision of approximately 5 cm in length using a wound protector in order to minimize the risk of tumor cell seeding [9–11, 24–27]. The proximal edge of the colon, which should reach the pelvis without tension, is pulled out of the peritoneal cavity through the wound protector, and its staple line at its edge is divided. An anvil is introduced into the lumen of the colon and fixed to its place using a purse string suture. The proximal edge is placed back in the peritoneal cavity, and the incision is closed in layers in order for the pneumoperitoneum to be reestablished. The circular stapler is inserted into the rectum transanally. The rectal stump is perforated with the spike of the circular stapler at its proximal edge. The anvil at the lower edge of the colon is attached to the spike at the upper edge of the rectum, taking into consideration not to twist the colon and the mesocolon (Fig. 2.22). The circular stapler is fired, creating the anastomosis. Subsequently, it is twisted open and removed through the anus [9–11, 24–31, 33]. The integrity of the anastomosis is confirmed by checking the integrity of the proximal and distal rings removed by the circular

Fig. 2.22 Making an
end-to-end colorectal
anastomosis with a
circular stapler

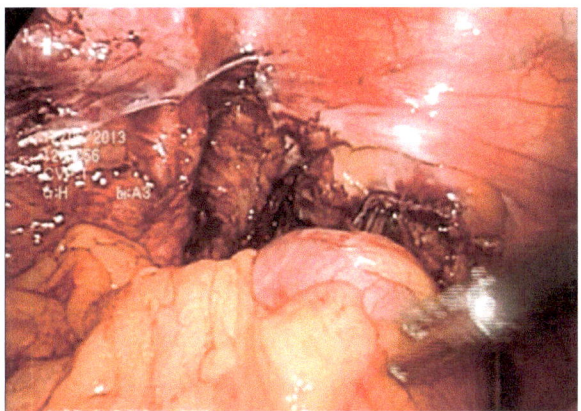

stapler and performing an air test. During the air test, the pelvis is filled with natural saline and air is insufflated into the rectum using a syringe or a rectoscope, while the bowel is gently occluded proximally to the anastomosis. A leak is confirmed if bubbles appear [9–11, 19, 24–29, 31]. If the air test is negative, the operation proceeds to its end. The peritoneal cavity is irrigated, the mesocolic defects are closed with interrupted sutures, and a drain may be placed at the site of anastomosis. The cannula sites are checked for bleeding, and the pneumoperitoneum and the cannulas are removed. The wounds are closed [9–11, 24–27].

2.5   Laparoscopic Subtotal Colectomy

There are several benign and malignant conditions, including ulcerative colitis, Crohn's disease, polyposis syndromes, lower gastro-intestinal hemorrhage, colonic cancer, and others that indicate subtotal colectomy as the procedure of choice in order to get the proper treatment. Usually, the population needing that type of surgery is young and the laparoscopic approach gives them the opportunity of a better cosmesis as well as the potential of another laparoscopic surgical procedure in the future. The operative technique is more or less a combination of right and left hemicolectomy described previously, so we are providing a short reference for the reader, from Ianelli A., who presented his own a few years ago. We place the patient in a supine lithotomy position with the limps abducted in order to avoid interference with the surgical instruments, while the arms are resting parallel to the trunk. We have already inserted both a nasogastric tube and a urine catheter, prior to any incision. After inserting a Veress needle, we induct the pneumoperitoneum and we insert a 10 mm port in the umbilicus for the 30° camera. Thereinafter two 5-mm and a 12 mm trocars are inserted with direct vision in both the upper quadrants and the right lower quadrant, respectively. As we have previously described, we proceed with soft tissue and mesocolon dissection, as well as vascular divisions including the inferior mesenteric artery, middle and superior right colic arteries, and superior rectal pedicles. Beginning from the right colon, keeping precisely in Toldt's plane, we dissect cecum and ascending colon, and we mobilize the ileocecal pedicle in order to divide it. We mobilize the hepatic flexure, we separate the gastrocolic ligament, and going to the left we mobilize the splenic flexure as well. We divide the vessels to the transverse colon, as well as the inferior mesenteric vessels at their origin. We perform the same mobilization for the left colon after the identification of the left ureter, in Toldt's plane as well. Afterwards, we divide the superior rectal pedicle and with a laparoscopic linear stapler, we transect the rectum just on the level of the sacral promontory leaving behind an adequate rectal stump [34]. Having all the specimen free, we perform a short incision in the right lower fossa in order to extract it from the peritoneal cavity, and ileo-rectum anastomosis is performed after the reestablishment of the pneumoperitoneum.

2.6   Laparoscopic Hartmann's Procedure and Hartmann's Reversal

Nowadays, the indications to perform a Hartmann colectomy are very limited, and can be implemented in urgent surgical situations, such as complicated diverticulitis, or obstructive ileus with extensive bowel dilatation and ischemia, wherein a colectomy and primary anastomosis are compromised. In those situations, taking into consideration the difficulties that follow that conditions, including the friable of the bowel wall, as well as the inflammatory changes to the mesentery, we should attempt a laparoscopic approach, with exactly the same surgical technique following in left colectomy/sigmoidectomy, sparing the final part of the anastomosis, with the creation of a left-sided end colostomy. At this point, it is essential to mention that concerning mobilization, specimen size, and number of lymph node removed, in cases of malignancy, we should make the effort to achieve the same oncological outcome as in scheduled colectomies.

An even more challenging laparoscopic operation is the reversal of a Hartmann procedure in order to restitute the colon continuance. Mainly there are two prevalent approaches depending on the attending doctor choice. Placed the patient in a lithotomy position, we either enter the peritoneal cavity from an optical-access trocar situated in the right upper abdomen, trying to be away from the previous incision and afterwards we insert two or three additional ports in the previous skin incisions, or we start the procedure with mobilization of the stoma from the skin. In the first approach, we start with the adhesiolysis at the colostomy site, we dissect the colostomy stoma detaching it from the abdominal wall in order to insert the anvil of a circular stapling devise into the proximal colon, suture the colostomy site, and restore pneumoperitoneum [35]. If we decide to begin from the stoma site, we mobilize the colostomy and at the end we use the stoma site as the port site for the establishment of the pneumoperitoneum. We mobilize the splenic flexure and the lateral attachments in order to ensure that we obtain an appropriate length of descending colon for a tension-free anastomosis with the rectal stump if this has not been performed previously. If we have difficulties recognizing the rectal stump, we can insert the stapling device or a bowel dilator transanally [35]. With the integrity of the anastomosis confirmed, the operation proceeds to its end.

2.7   Laparoscopic Low Anterior Colectomy and Abdominoperineal Resection

Even though the laparoscopic treatment of rectal cancer is beyond the scope of this chapter, especially because of the differences that exist either in oncological or in confrontational point of view, we have the ambition to provide to the readers a short reference concerning this particular surgical entity.

Over the last decades, we have noticed an ongoing improvement in oncological outcomes of patients undergoing treatment for rectal cancer due to a multimodal treatment which compounds both adjuvant/neoadjuvant chemo-radiotherapy and total mesorectal excision (TME), with the last to play a significant role in the local recurrence rate as well as in the positive circumferential resection margin (CRM) rate. Additionally, according to many randomized clinical trials, we can achieve significant improvement in local control with the implementation of neoadjuvant treatment. From the surgical point of view, laparoscopic TME compared with the open approach is a technically feasible and safe operation with an oncological outcome similar between the two methods but with a great difference in terms of postoperative recovery and complications.

Both laparoscopic low anterior colectomy and abdominoperineal resection have almost the same patient and trocar placement, slightly different from the left colectomy or sigmoidectomy presented above, with a medial to lateral dissection method (Fig. 2.23).

The main difference and distinguish characteristic is the implementation of TME regardless of the type of operation performed in order to achieve the

Fig. 2.23 Trocar placement for low anterior resection [7]

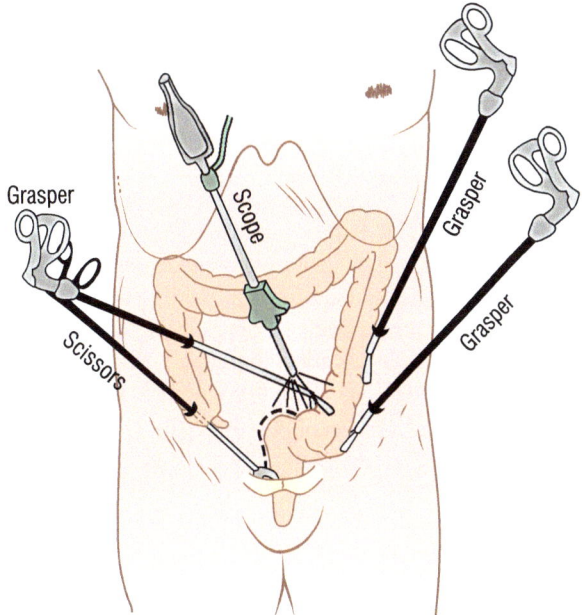

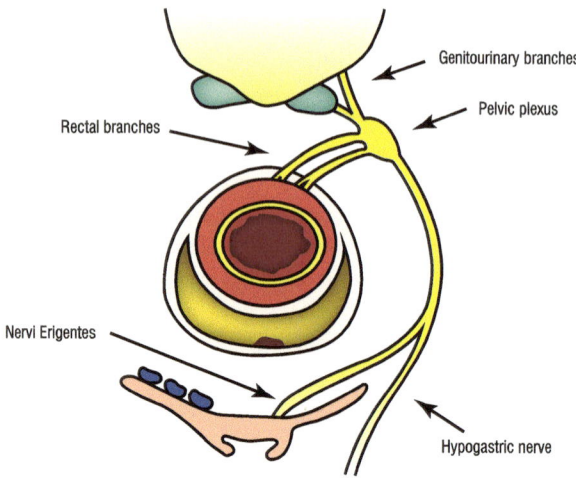

Fig. 2.24 Schematic view of the anatomy of the pelvic nerves and plexi [36]

optimal therapeutic result, as well as the final step of the abdominoperineal resection, since we have to resect the anal sphincter complex using both anterior abdominal approach and perineal incision, resulting in a permanent colostomy, instead of an anastomosis. In regard to the vascular approach and colon mobilization, we follow the same steps mentioned above for left hemicolectomy. TME must be performed with special consideration to identify and preserve the pelvic autonomic plexus, as well as the left and right hypogastric nerves and consider as completed when we have reached the pelvic floor (levators) first posteriorly, then laterally, and finally by approaching the anterior plane (Fig. 2.24) [36]. The anterior resection begins at the level of peritoneal reflection with an upside down U-line incision.

The main and significant point at this time is to maintain a permanent cephalad retraction of the upper rectum in order to achieve an easily identifiable plan. While we have incorporated the peritoneal reflection dissection and the lower rectum has been revealed, we identify the seminal vesicles, having a prominent tubular presentation. Then we proceed along the Denonvilliers' fascia in men or the rectovaginal septum in women. At this point (in men), we can identify the characteristic smooth posterior border of the prostate gland. Along this dissection, we have to identify the periprostatic plexus that contains both sympathetic and parasympathetic fibers in order to avoid postoperative complications such as incomplete erection, problems in ejaculation or even complete impotence. When we have achieved an adequate mobilization of the rectum and we have defined the distal resection line for the low anterior colectomy, we grasp the bowel either with a right angle clamp or with a linear stapler in order to isolate the lumen distal to the pathology. In case of an abdominoperineal resection, after the completion of the TME, we have to mobilize the anal sphincter complex below the pelvic floor with either an intersphincteric or an extrasphincteric plane [37, 38].

2.8 Laparoscopic Colectomy in an Obese Patient

Even though the advantages of laparoscopic procedures are undoubtable, there are some issues concerning laparoscopic colectomies that may lead to surgical difficulties. The major problems become apparent due to the obesity of the patient. In general, obese patients benefit from laparoscopy. Many laparoscopic procedures, such as cholecystectomy, hernias, Nissen fundoplication, sleeve gastrectomy, gastric bypass, and many others have found major applications, or are applied especially for obese patients. On the other hand, laparoscopy in obese patients may have a negative impact in the ability of the technique, or results to an increase duration of the procedure and blood lose. At this point, we are aware that this special group of patients have particular issues concerning open surgery such as extended incisions for better visualization and bowel mobilization and increased minor or major postsurgical complications. On the contrary with the laparoscopic techniques, we have the ability to expand the surgical field with a minor intervention, such as the insertion of an extra trocar, or to achieve substantial decrease in complications occurred.

Through a nice and systematic literature research, Hana Alhomoud published a relevant review article in order to point out potential differences or superiority between open and laparoscopic colectomy. She concluded that the existing evidence suggests that laparoscopy in obese patients for colorectal diseases does not increase mortality or reoperation rates and does not result in worst recovery or intestinal malfunction. In most of the studies that she included in her review, it was apparent that even longer operation times or higher conversion rates have no influence in the feasibility or the curative result of the technique [39].

References

1. Siegel R, Ma J, Zou Z, et al. Cancer statistics, 2014. CA Cancer J Clin. 2014;64:9–29.
2. Ding J, Xia Y, Zhang ZM, et al. Laparoscopic versus open right hemicolectomy for colon cancer: a meta- analysis. J Laparoendosc Adv Surg Tech A. 2013;23:8–16.
3. Lacy AM, García-Valdecasas JC, Delgado S, et al. Laparoscopy-assisted colectomy versus open colectomy for treatment of non-metastatic colon cancer: a randomised trial. Lancet. 2002;359:2224–9.
4. Nelson H. A comparison of laparoscopically assisted and open colectomy for colon cancer. N Engl J Med. 2004;350:2050–9.
5. Welch CE, Ottinger LW, Welch JP. Anatomy and physiology of the colon and rectum. In: Manual of lower gastrointestinal surgery. New York: Springer; 1980. p. 9–18.
6. Milsom JW, Böhm B, Nakajima K. Laparoscopic anatomy of the abdominal cavity. In: Laparoscopic colorectal surgery. 2nd ed. New York, NY: Springer; 2006. p. 97–110.
7. Skandalakis LJ, Skandalakis JE. Colon and anorectum. In: Skandalakis LJ, Skandalakis JE, editors. Surgical anatomy and technique: a pocket manual. 4th ed. New York, NY: Springer; 2014. p. 431–514.
8. Branum GD, Pappas TN. Laparoscopic-assisted colectomy and abdominoperineal resection. In: Atlas of laparoscopic surgery. New York, NY: Springer; 1996. p. 193–202.
9. Milsom JW, Bohm B. Laparoscopic colorectal surgery. New York: Springer Verlag; 1996.
10. Leroy J, Henri M, Rubino F, Marescaux J. Sigmoidectomy. In: Laparoscopic colorectal surgery. 2nd ed. New York, NY: Springer; 2006. p. 145–69.

11. Pendlimari R, Nelson H. Laparoscopic colorectal procedures. In: Maingot's abdominal operations. 12th ed. New York, NY: The McGraw-Hill Companies; 2013. p. 767–94.
12. Marchesi F, Pinna F, Percalli L, Cecchini S, Riccó M, Costi R, Pattonieri V, Roncoroni L. Totally laparoscopic right colectomy: theoretical and practical advantages over the laparo-assisted approach. J Laparoendosc Adv Surg Tech A. 2013;23(5):418–24.
13. Goasguen N, Mosnier H. Laparoscopic right colectomy. J Visc Surg. 2010;147(1):e41–6.
14. Dimitriou N, Griniatsos J. Complete mesocolic excision: techniques and outcomes. World J Gastrointest Oncol. 2015;7(12):383–8.
15. Vergis AS, Steigerwald SN, Bhojani FD, Sullivan PA, Hardy KM. Laparoscopic right hemicolectomy with intracorporeal versus extracorporeal anastomosis: a comparison of short-term outcomes. Can J Surg. 2015;58(1):63–8.
16. Chang K, Fakhoury M, Barnajian M, Tarta C, Bergamaschi R. Laparoscopic right colon resection with intracorporeal anastomosis. Surg Endosc. 2013;27(5):1730–6.
17. Roscio F, Bertoglio C, De Luca A, Frattini P, Scandroglio I. Totally laparoscopic versus laparoscopic assisted right colectomy for cancer. Int J Surg. 2012;10(6):290–5.
18. Ho YH. Laparoscopic right hemicolectomy with intracorporeal anastomosis. Tech Coloproctol. 2010;14(4):359–63.
19. O'Mahoney PR, Trencheva K, Zhuo C, Shukla PJ, Lee SW, Sonoda T, Milsom JW. Systematic video documentation in laparoscopic colon surgery using a checklist: a feasibility and compliance pilot study. J Laparoendosc Adv Surg Tech A. 2015;25(9):737–43.
20. Haas EM, Pedraza R, Nieto J, Malave V. Single-incision laparoscopic right hemicolectomy: inferior-to-superior approach with intracorporeal anastomosis. Surg Laparosc Endosc Percutan Tech. 2014;24(6):e226–7.
21. Erguner I, Aytac E, Baca B, Hamzaoglu I, Karahasanoglu T. Total laparoscopic approach for the treatment of right colon cancer: a technical critique. Asian J Surg. 2013;36(2):58–63.
22. Wong JT, Abbas MA. Laparoscopic right hemicolectomy. Tech Coloproctol. 2013;17(Suppl 1):S3–9.
23. Levard H, Denet C, Gayet B. Laparoscopic right colectomy from top to bottom. J Visc Surg. 2012;149(1):e34–7.
24. Monson J. Technique of laparoscopic left hemicolectomy. Int J Surg Investig. 1999;1(3):249–50.
25. Zucker KA. Laparoscopic left hemicolectomy and sigmoidectomy. In: Laparoscopic surgery of the abdomen. New York, NY: Springer; 2004. p. 369–79.
26. Young-Fadok TM. Laparoscopic left hemicolectomy. In: Fischer's mastery of surgery. 6th ed. Philadelphia, PA: Lippincott Williams & Wilkins; 2012. p. 1655–60.
27. Ricciardi K, Wexner SD. Laparoscopic left hemicolectomy and low anterior resection. In: Chassin's operative strategy in general surgery. 4th ed. New York, NY: Springer; 2014. p. 489–500.
28. Huang CC, Chen YC, Huang CJ, Hsieh JS. Totally laparoscopic colectomy with intracorporeal side-to- end colorectal anastomosis and transrectal specimen extraction for sigmoid and rectal cancers. Ann Surg Oncol. 2016;23(4):1164–8.
29. Colombo PE, Rouanet P. Laparoscopic left colectomy for cancer. J Visc Surg. 2010;147(5):e297–304.
30. Akamatsu H, Omori T, Oyama T, Tori M, Ueshima S, Nakahara M, Abe T, Nishida T. Totally laparoscopic sigmoid colectomy: a simple and safe technique for intracorporeal anastomosis. Surg Endosc. 2009;23(11):2605–59.
31. Lee SW, Yoo J, Dujovny N, Sonoda T, Milsom JW. Laparoscopic vs. hand-assisted laparoscopic sigmoidectomy for diverticulitis. Dis Colon Rectum. 2006;49(4):464–9.
32. Swaid F, Sroka G, Madi H, Shteinberg D, Somri M, Matter I. Totally laparoscopic versus laparoscopic- assisted left colectomy for cancer: a retrospective review. Surg Endosc. 2016;30(6):2481–8.
33. Bucher P, Wutrich P, Pugin F, Gonzales M, Gervaz P, Morel P. Totally intracorporeal laparoscopic colorectal anastomosis using circular stapler. Surg Endosc. 2008;22(5):1278–82.
34. Iannelli A, Fabiani P, Mouiel J, et al. Laparoscopic subtotal colectomy with cecorectal anastomosis for slow-transit constipation. Surg Endosc. 2006;20:171–3.

35. Park J-M, Chi K-C. Laparoscopic reversal of Hartmann's procedure. J Korean Surg Soc. 2012;82(4):256–60.
36. Masaro S, Palmisano S, Leon P, de Manzini N. Nerve- sparing technique in rectal cancer. Strategy and Surgical Techniques, Springer: In Rectal Cancer; 2013. p. 107–15.
37. Palanivelu C, Sendhilkumar K, Kalpesh J, et al. Laparoscopic anterior resection and total mesorectal excision for rectal cancer: a prospective nonrandomized study. Int J Color Dis. 2007;22:367–72.
38. Wang YW, Huang LY, Song CL, et al. Laparoscopic vs open abdominoperineal resection in the multimodality management of low rectal cancers. World J Gastroenterol. 2015;21(35):10174–83.
39. Alhomoud H. The impact of obesity in laparoscopic colorectal resection. World J Laparosc Surg. 2013;6(3):144–8.

Preoperative Evaluation and Selection of Patients

Konstantinos Bramis and George Bagias

3.1 Introduction

Minimal invasive surgery is consistently gaining ground since its introduction in the 1980s, as it has many perioperative and postoperative advantages over conventional surgery, such as less intraoperative bleeding, less postoperative pain, shorter hospitalization, and smaller wounds with lower incidence for incisional hernias; these make minimal invasive procedures the standard approach for many operations. Since 1991, when Jacobs et al. introduced laparoscopic colon resection [1], a tremendous progress has been made so that today laparoscopic colorectal surgery is much accepted as a safe and feasible surgical technique. Improvements in technology have led to the adoption of new technical modifications, which allow the use of laparoscopy in both benign pathologies and colon carcinomas.

However, the eligible patients for laparoscopic colon surgery should be selected carefully, as not all cases are suitable for laparoscopy; some cases should be primarily operated conventionally. In this chapter, the authors attempt to analyze thoroughly the preoperative evaluation and selection of patients who should undergo a laparoscopic colorectal operation and they discuss the indications and contraindications of each surgical approach.

K. Bramis (✉)
Aretaieio Hospital of Athens, National and Kapodistrian University of Athens, Athens, Greece

G. Bagias
1st Propaedeutic Surgical Department, Hippokration Hospital, University of Athens, Athens, Greece

3.2 General Indications and Contraindications for Laparoscopic Surgery

In general, laparoscopic surgery is associated with less surgical trauma and faster postoperative recovery; both are factors that can influence the incidence of early and late postoperative complications. Numerous large randomized studies have highlighted the superiority of laparoscopy in colon surgery in terms of early postoperative course [2, 3]. Comparing patients who were operated conventionally with patients who underwent open surgery, patients after laparoscopic colon resection had lower incidence of postoperative anemia because of less intraoperative blood loss, fewer postoperative cardiopulmonary complications, earlier and faster normalization of the bowel motility, and decreased rate of surgical wound infections [2–4]. Consequently, patients who underwent a laparoscopic colon resection could be discharged earlier. Interestingly, laparoscopic surgery in elder patients can be associated with better survival rates mainly because of the shorter and less complicated postoperative course [5]. Long-term outcomes of laparoscopic colorectal surgery are also superior to those of open surgery. Various meta-analyses that compared minimal invasive to traditional surgery showed a higher 1-year, 3-year, and consecutive 5-year survival rate in colorectal cancer patients [5, 6]. In terms of oncological outcomes, laparoscopic colon resection is comparable to open surgery. In a recent meta-analysis, there was no statistically significant difference in disease-free survival and overall survival rate between laparoscopic and open surgery for low rectal cancer [7].

Although its short- and long-term outcomes are unquestionable, laparoscopic colorectal surgery has not yet been adopted broadly yet. To date, laparoscopic colorectal operations are performed only in 20–35% of all cases worldwide. Only in reference, high-volume centers this percentage raises to a maximum of 45% [4, 8–10]. Most surgeons support that the underlying pathology is the primary reason of choosing one technique versus the other. It is generally believed that in technically difficult operations, surgeons prefer the open technique. Difficult cases are colon carcinoma, larger in size and advanced in stage tumors, and tumors at inconvenient location, which are difficult to access [10]. Other factors that influence a surgeon's decision to follow a certain surgical technique against another are the patient's age, the American Society of Anesthesiologists' Risk Classification (ASA) status (shown in Appendix 3.1), the patient's body mass index (BMI), and the urgent nature of the operation [10].

To date, laparoscopy is the method of choice in elective cases to treat younger patients with benign conditions, with an ASA score of I or II, or at a low tumor stage. On the contrary, more challenging cases, such as advanced tumors with lymphatic spread or difficult to access tumor location at the right or left flexure, are usually treated with laparotomy. Although laparoscopic colorectal surgery has similar oncological results with open surgery and, as we mentioned above, survival rate is better in patients who were operated laparoscopically, open surgery is mostly chosen mainly because of the tough learning curve of laparoscopic colectomy and the difficulty of acquiring the necessary surgical skills. Moreover, in a study from

Marks et al., (2008), it was shown that high-risk patients could potentially benefit the most from a laparoscopic approach because of smaller trauma and faster postoperative course [11]. As far as factors related to surgeons' capabilities are concerned, surgeon's age, previous laparoscopic training, dexterity, and experience influence their decision of selecting patients who will be operated laparoscopically. Other factors, such as academic affiliation, lack of available operative time, and patient's insurance status, play an important role in patient selection. Finally, a colorectal operation during the night shift is more likely to be performed conventionally, as the surgical staff in charge is not always trained to minimal invasive colon operations [10]. Furthermore, the majority of the cases that need to be operated during the night shift are on an emergency basis (e.g., colon perforation, colonic obstruction), where minimal invasive approach is not recommended.

A strong argument against laparoscopic colorectal surgery has to do with the cost of the procedure; laparoscopic colectomy might require more time to be performed compared to the conventional, open technique. Also, laparoscopic instruments are expensive and most of them are for single use, something that increases their cost further. To counterfeit this, other experts argue that because of less postoperative complications, fewer reoperations and readmissions, and fewer days of hospitalization, the total cost of laparoscopic colorectal treatment is lower compared to the total cost of the open surgical treatment.

Experience has proven that as surgical skills are improved and as the cost of training becomes more effective, the total operative cost of laparoscopic colectomy can become similar or less than the operative cost of the open colon surgery.

3.3 Special Considerations

In the previous paragraphs, we highlighted the superiority of laparoscopic colorectal surgery in terms of perioperative and early postoperative morbidity. Although this surgical technique is considered safe and feasible, not all patients with colon pathology will eventually undergo a laparoscopic colon resection. Among the factors mentioned above who may influence the surgical decision towards laparoscopy, there are also disease-related factors, which should be also considered before choosing the right approach to follow. Usually, the more severe and complex a disease is, the more likely is the operation to be performed conventionally.

Herein, we analyze the preoperative evaluation of patients with the most common surgical pathologies of the colon, which factors are indicative of a surgical therapy, and how the surgeons determine when they will perform laparoscopic colon surgery.

3.3.1 Inflammatory Bowel Disease

Treatment of the inflammatory bowel diseases (IBD) has changed during the last decades. Current conservative medical therapy is able to suppress disease's progression for a long time, yet a large number of patients with IBD will be eventually in need of surgery. Surgical treatment of IBD includes large colon resections with permanent postoperative outcomes, impairing postoperative quality of life. Therefore, the adoption of minimal invasive approach is essential for this population of patients, as it can improve outcomes and quality of life after surgery. However, laparoscopic colorectal surgery for IBD is challenging, as many technical difficulties arise because of its pathophysiology; hence, the selection of patients who should undergo a laparoscopic procedure should be made carefully.

3.3.1.1 Crohn's Disease

Crohn's disease (CD) is an inflammatory bowel disease which can actually be present throughout the gastrointestinal tract. During the past years, conservative medical therapy has significantly increased efficacy of disease control, yet about 60–70% of all CD patients will be finally operated for disease's complications, such as stricture, abscess, fistula, hemorrhage, malnutrition, and/or tumor [12]. In addition, about 60% of the cases operated will develop disease recurrence and in 30% of them a reoperation will be needed, which can be very challenging because of the intra-abdominal adhesions that might have developed after the first surgery [12]. Other factors that may lead to surgery CD patients are the thick and friable inflammatory mesentery and the high risk of postoperative complications that can be augmented after medical therapy.

CD patients are usually young, fit, with low BMI index and facts such as smaller trauma and shorter postoperative course are essential to them. Therefore, despite its technical difficulties, minimal invasive colorectal surgery has a place in the treatment of CD. The terminal ileum is the most affected site in CD patients and complications such as stricture or abscess indicate ileocolic resection. In uncomplicated cases of CD (absence of fistula and/or intra-abdominal adhesions), the use of laparoscopy is strongly recommended. In patients with CD, however, hybrid approaches such as laparoscopic-assisted or hand-assisted laparoscopic surgery are preferred, as technical difficulties may arise due to inflamed bowel mesentery. Moreover, a thorough exploration of the abdomen for detection of unknown strictures or occult segments is also needed.

In hand-assisted technique, a 5 cm incision is performed, allowing the insertion of the surgeon's hand, facilitating the laparoscopic dissection, while exploring the rest bowel to rule out other sites of disease. In the laparoscopic-assisted hybrid procedure, the dissection is performed totally laparoscopically and the anastomosis is performed extracorporeally. Laparoscopic ileocolic resection is safe and feasible, with a conversion rate of about 2% [13]. However, there are certain factors in patients with CD that are associated with higher risk for conversion. Smoking, treatment with steroid or with immunosuppressive agents, extracecal colonic disease, and preoperative malnutrition are predicting factors for conversion.

In patients with uncomplicated CD, laparoscopy should still be performed. However, in cases where an intra-abdominal fistula or abscess is present, or an additional colon segment should be simultaneously resected, surgeons should consider the open technique as the procedure of choice. This recommendation applies also in cases of recurrent CD, where the risk of conversion is also high; it approaches 40% [13].

In terms of postoperative morbidity, laparoscopic ileocecal resection seems to have lower morbidity rate, faster postoperative course, and better pulmonary and bowel function recovery. Recurrence rate is similar between the two approaches, implying that laparoscopic exploration is adequate and comparable to open approach, when it is performed by experienced surgeons. Last but not least, with laparoscopy, wound scars are smaller or even invisible, giving better aesthetic results, which is much appreciated by patients.

Crohn's colitis occurs in about 10% of patients with CD. Patients with severe acute colitis, which may be refractory to medical therapy, should be selected for surgical treatment [14]. To date, acute colitis complicated with perforation, massive hemorrhage, or megacolon is treated with open procedure and laparoscopy is contraindicated. However, acute colitis, without the complications mentioned above, can be treated with subtotal colectomy, which can be performed laparoscopically. Yet, a Hartmann's procedure, applying an end colostomy is strongly recommended, and primary reconstruction of the colon should be avoided, as the risk for anastomotic insufficiency in this population is high (long-term steroid medication, preoperative malnutrition).

Although there are only few large series and meta-analyses studies comparing laparoscopic and open subtotal colectomy, laparoscopic surgical treatment seems to be safe and feasible. Postoperative morbidity rate after laparoscopy is the same or even lower compared to the open surgery. Furthermore, postoperative recovery and total length of stay are lower after laparoscopy. Nevertheless, laparoscopic subtotal colectomy is a challenging procedure, with significantly longer operative time and conversion rate that ranges between 11% and 26% [13]; only surgeons trained in laparoscopic surgery should carry out such a procedure, and preferably not on an emergency basis.

3.3.1.2 Ulcerative Colitis
Ulcerative colitis (UC) is an inflammatory bowel disease characterized by chronic mucosal and submucosal inflammation, which is confined to colon and rectum. Like Crohn's disease, a large number of patients with UC will be eventually in need of surgical treatment. Failure of medical treatment is the most common indication for surgery. Patients in acute phase of UC who are under intravenous steroid therapy and have a stool frequency of more than eight times per day or a CRP higher than 45 mg/L are considered candidates for surgery [15]. Additionally, presence of refractory UC, despite initial response to conservative treatment, is also an indication for an operative therapy. In a chronic set, 5–30% of patients with UC will experience malignant transformation, which is an absolute indication for surgery. Dysplasia sites in large intestinal mucosal biopsies can be initially removed endoscopically; however, when the dysplastic tissue cannot be removed totally or when multifocal dysplasia is discovered, a surgical treatment should be considered. Some authors support that high-grade dysplasia alone can be an indication for operative treatment because the risk of underlying malignancy is up to 40%. Severe

complications of UC, such as toxic megacolon, perforation, and hemorrhage, are absolute, yet, rare indications for surgery.

To date, total proctocolectomy and ileal pouch–anal anastomosis (IPAA) are the procedures of choice for patients with UC. Recent large studies and meta-analyses have shown that advanced age is not a contraindication for IPAA, as postoperative complications and pouch preservation rates are not correlated with patient age, although it is true that pouch function deteriorates faster in elder patients.

Concerns have been aroused for IPAA, though, when the diagnosis of UC is unclear; in 10–15% of patients after subtotal colectomy on an emergency case, histopathological examination cannot differentiate between UC and CD [16]. These patients have consistently good results from IPAA surgery. Nevertheless, the incidence of pelvic sepsis and pouch failure is higher in this group of patients. Thus, an IPAA procedure is not contraindicated when the diagnosis is unclear, but the patient should be thoroughly informed about the possible risks.

Laparoscopic-assisted proctocolectomy with IPAA was first described in 1992, yet its use is still questionable. After early disappointing results, large case series comparing laparoscopic and open approach were published. Generally, postoperative morbidity, postoperative length of stay, and quality of life are not statistically significant better in patients who underwent laparoscopy, and the operating room time, for the laparoscopic surgical treatment, is significantly longer than open surgery. However, some authors proposed that, although it is not statistically significant, postoperative recovery is faster in patients after laparoscopic proctocolectomy, with lower incidence of septic complications, anastomotic leakage and postoperative bowel obstruction, blood loss, and mortality. Long-term outcomes after laparoscopic-assisted proctocolectomy are also not better compared to those after open procedure; in a Cochrane review of 607 patients from 12 studies, no significant differences in complications, readmission, reoperation rates, and mortality rate were identified [17]. Nevertheless, the key advantage of laparoscopic proctocolectomy is the cosmetic result, which is essential for many patients.

To conclude, laparoscopic proctocolectomy should be performed only by experienced surgeons on selected cases of non-fulminant UC.

3.3.2   Endometriosis

Endometriosis is one of the most common benign, but refractory gynecological diseases, as it affects 7–10% of women of reproductive age [18]. Endometriomas can be found inter alia in peritoneum, in ovaries, and in rectovaginal septum, which is called deep endometriosis (DE). Deep endometriosis of the intestine occurs in 8–12% of women with endometriosis and mostly (90%) affects the colon and the rectum [18]. Patients with DE are experiencing dysmenorrhea, dyspareunia, noncyclic pelvic pain, infertility, as well as specific bowel symptoms such as hematochezia and cyclic bowel alterations. Patients with rectal endometriosis can even have cyclic defecation pain and cyclic constipation, leading to bowel obstruction. However, the severity of symptoms may not reflect size and extend of the lesions;

therefore, a surgical intervention should not be based only on the intensity of the symptoms. Patients should be operated when they have (a) significant pain such as dyspareunia and dyschezia, which impairs life quality or (b) signs of bowel obstruction. Moreover, a surgical intervention should be considered when women with DE, who wish to have children, had at least two failed in vitro fertilization (IVF) cycles.

The main objective of surgery for DE is the complete excision of all endometriotic lesions. To date, there are three different procedures used in the treatment of DE: (a) the shaving technique, where the endometrioma is locally excised or ablated, (b) disk resection of the endometriotic nodule, where the endometrioma is completely resected from colon/rectum followed by closure of bowel wall, and (c) segmental resection with end-to-end anastomosis, where the colon segment, which consists the endometrioma, is completely resected, followed by the anastomosis of the proximal and distal colon segment. The choice of surgical procedure depends on anatomical and histological features of DE. First, when an endometriotic lesion infiltrates the inner layer of muscularis propria or gets deeper, it should be radically removed with segmental resection, as the circumference of the bowel affected by the disease is higher than 40% and possible disk resection will lead to postoperative stenosis. When it infiltrates the outer layer of muscularis propria or serosa, other factors should be taken into consideration. One of them is the number of endometriotic lesions. Multifocality is not rare in rectovaginal DE; approximately 40% of patients with rectovaginal DE have more than two lesions across a colon segment. Also, in this case, a segmental resection should be performed, followed by end-to-end anastomosis. Another factor is the lesion's size. Endometriomas larger than 3 cm in diameter require a segmental resection to avoid significant distortion of the bowel axis and subsequent stricture. A superficial lesion can, regardless of its size, be removed through shaving, keeping in mind, though, the risk of disease recurrence, while for nodules smaller than 3 cm, a discoid resection can also be considered. Finally, in cases of advanced DE, a lymphadenectomy should be performed, as the disease can be disseminated to lymph nodes causing a disease recurrence. Prognostic factors for lymphatic dissemination are the size of the bowel lesion and the percentage of the intestinal wall. Nowadays, all three procedures are performed mostly laparoscopically. All procedures are associated with relatively low postoperative morbidity (1–15%) and better quality of life postoperatively. Recurrence rate is low and when a segmental resection is performed, recurrence rate is below 20%.

3.3.3 Diverticulitis

Diverticular disease ranges from an asymptomatic diverticular disease to acute, perforated diverticulitis. Diverticulitis is defined as an inflammation of one or more diverticula, which can potentially lead to perforation. As a result, not all patients with acute diverticulitis will be finally treated surgically. The Hinchey's classification for proper preoperative evaluation and selection of patients was introduced, which classifies acute diverticulitis into four stages according to clinical presentation and imaging findings (Table 3.1). Stage I diverticulitis is defined as the

Table 3.1 Hinchey's classification of acute diverticulitis

Stage	Description
I	Diverticulitis with phlegmon (1a) or localized abscess (1b)
II	Diverticulitis with retroperitoneal and/or pelvic abscess
III	Diverticulitis with generalized purulent peritonitis
IV	Diverticulitis with generalized faecal peritonitis

inflammation of usually one diverticulum, with phlegmon, or localized pericolic, or mesenteric abscess. Stage II diverticulitis is associated with walled off pelvic, intra-abdominal, or retroperitoneal abscess. In Stage III diverticulitis, the inflammation coexists along with perforation of the diverticulum, causing generalized purulent peritonitis. Finally, in Stage IV diverticulitis, the diverticulum is ruptured into the peritoneal cavity with fecal contamination causing generalized fecal peritonitis.

As we mentioned before, only a small number of patients with acute diverticulitis will be operated on an emergency basis. Patients with acute diverticulitis without perforation will be treated with the appropriate medical treatment. When conservative therapy fails, surgical treatment should be chosen. Of those who were successfully treated conservatively, about 30% will undergo an elective sigmoidectomy in the future. It is generally accepted that patients after the second course of, an otherwise uncomplicated, diverticulitis should be operated. Although this statement is popular, the indication for surgery should be rather patient-related, evaluating patient's ASA score and quality of life. It is also believed that younger patients should be eventually operated, as they tend to have more episodes of diverticulitis during their life. This statement is true, yet disease recurrence is not associated with age. Therefore, patient's age alone cannot indicate a surgical treatment.

According to recent guidelines, an elective resection is indicated in recurrent diverticulitis with significant impairment of quality of life. Moreover, an elective sigmoid resection, 6–8 weeks after recovery from a covert perforated diverticulitis, should also be considered. A concealed perforation leads to persistent histologic alteration of the large intestine, which can lead to recurrence or persistent symptoms. In addition, *World Society of Emergency Surgery* recommends an elective sigmoid resection in patients with Stage II diverticulitis with pelvic abscess, because this subgroup of patients tends to develop disease recurrence more frequently compared to mesocolic abscesses [19]. Moreover, it is suggested that patients under immunosuppression should undergo an elective surgery after an episode of uncomplicated acute diverticulitis as prophylaxis; same is suggested for transplanted patients. However, this last suggestion remains until today controversial, as a limited number of studies have examined the prophylactic role of sigmoidectomy in this subgroup of patients.

Nevertheless, the role of laparoscopy in elective surgery is unquestionable. Laparoscopic sigmoidectomy is safe, feasible, with comparable morbidity to open procedure, although it is associated with longer operating time. It is also correlated with less postoperative pain and shorter hospitalization. Long-term outcomes regarding symptoms management and disease recurrence do not differ significantly between the two approaches, yet patients who underwent laparoscopic sigmoidectomy refer better quality of life. The role of surgery in acute complicated diverticulitis (Hinchey III and IV) is beyond doubt. An explorative laparotomy is still the most common approach, though all updated guidelines underline the role of minimal invasive approach in management of acute complicated diverticulitis as the standard approach, except Stage IV diverticulitis, where an open procedure should be followed. It is generally recommended that a laparoscopic lavage, with bowel resection and without bowel reconstruction, should be performed on an emergency basis. A second operation is performed 24–48 h after and it is decided whether a primary anastomosis or Hartmann's procedure should be followed. This strategy allows better sepsis control and is correlated with lower rate of anastomotic insufficiency. All recent guidelines conclude that a Hartmann's procedure should be avoided if possible; although it is a safe procedure, it resolves into permanent bowel discontinuity, because in 40% of all patients the terminal colostomy will not be reversed, impairing patient's life quality.

3.3.4 Benign Tumors

Colorectal adenomas or adenomatous polyps have a high malignant potential; 4% of colorectal adenomas will transform in carcinomas after 5 years and this rate rises to 14% after 10 years. Nowadays, the quintessence of colorectal cancer prevention is the identification and eradication of these lesions. Polyps can be removed by using endoscopic, surgical, or combined methods. To date, most polyps are removed endoscopically, yet it has been reported that residual malignant disease (in the large intestine's wall or regional lymph nodes) can be as high as 39% in malignant polyps with unfavorable histology [20]. Nevertheless, about 10–15% of all colorectal polyps cannot be removed endoscopically due to their size, configuration, and location in the colon.

In cases of adenomas located in inconvenient sites, laparoscopically assisted colonoscopic polypectomy can be performed. Under laparoscopy, the part of the colon proximal to the lesion is clamped and mobilized, so that an endoscopic mucosectomy can be performed. This technique is safe, feasible, and quite efficient. When adenomas, mostly due to their size (size >7 cm), cannot be removed endoscopically, a colotomy with polypectomy, a segmental colon resection, or even a right/left hemicolectomy can be carried out. In this setting, laparoscopic surgery has a strong indication; patients are mostly young, fit, and they have a benign or borderline malignant disease and, therefore, will be benefited the most from laparoscopy. Elder patients can also be benefited from laparoscopic surgery; the postoperative course will be shorter, meaning less possibility for postoperative complications. However, if a malignant adenoma is suspected, an open procedure should be considered to master a formal oncologic resection with central vascular ligation and lymphadenectomy.

3.3.5   Malignant Tumors

Colorectal cancer is the third most common carcinoma in the Western world; yet thanks to the improvement of surgical and conventional management, the overall survival rate is up to 50%. To achieve the best oncological and survival outcomes, treatment strategy should be individualized and personalized. Like in every malignancy, thorough staging with colonoscopy, histological assessment of all lesions, and evaluation of images from computed tomography (CT) of the abdomen and pelvis are mandatory. Preoperative assessment of carcinoembryonic antigen should be made to identify residual disease or disease recurrence. For rectal tumors, an endorectal ultrasound or alternatively a high-resolution magnetic resonance imaging (MRI) should be also performed. The *TNM* system, as proposed from the International Union Against Cancer (UICC), should be used to determine tumor stage, depending on the depth of the local tumor invasion (*T* stage), the extend of regional lymph node involvement (*N* stage), and the presence of distant metastasis (*M* stage) [21] (Table 3.2).

The basic concept of colorectal cancer management is the surgical removal of the tumor; pretreatment tumor staging is crucial for planning the treatment strategy. Early stage colorectal tumors (Stage I, T1N0M0) can be excided locally in patients with severe comorbidities, who are medically unfit for radical surgery. When the tumor is completely (R0) resected and the histological analysis shows a well-differentiated tumor, then a watch-and-wait strategy is indicated. On the other hand,

Table 3.2   TNM classification of cancer of the colon and rectum [21]

Primary tumor (T)	
TX T0	Primary tumor cannot be assessed No evidence of primary tumor
Tis T1 T2 T3	Carcinoma in situ: invasion of lamina propria Tumor invades submucosa Tumor invades muscularis propria
T4	Tumor invades subserosa or into non peritonealized pericolic or perirectal tissues
T4a T4b	Tumor directly invades other organs or structures and/or perforates visceral peritoneum
Regional lymph nodes (N)	
NX N0 N1	Regional lymph nodes cannot be assessed N0 No regional lymph node metastasis Metastasis in 1 to 3 regional lymph nodes N1a Metastasis in 1 regional lymph node Metastasis in 2 to 3 regional lymph nodes
N1a N1b N1c	Tumor deposit(s), i.e. satellites, in the subserosa, or in non peritonealized pericolic or perirectal soft tissue without regional lymph node metastasis
N2	Metastasis in 4 or more regional lymph nodes Metastasis in 4–6 regional lymph nodes Metastasis in 7 or more regional lymph nodes
Distant metastasis (M)	
M0	No distant metastasis
M1	Distant metastasis
M1a	Metastasis confined to one organ (liver, lung, ovary, non regional lymph node(s)) without peritoneal metastases
M1b	Metastasis in more than one organ
M1c	Metastasis to the peritoneum with or without other organ involvement

in a less differentiated tumor or when there is presence of lymphatic invasion, surgical resection is the recommended treatment. Otherwise, a local or distant recurrence, through lymphatic spread, would be very likely to happen.

Apparently, when there is a resectable colon tumor with stage > T1N0 (Table 3.3), the oncologically optimal operation is a colectomy with free-from-tumor resection margins (R0), and en-bloc1 complete removal of the resected segment mesocolon (complete mesocolic excision—CME), with all the regional lymph nodes. Resection margins should be at least 10 cm, unless this is not technically efficient because of the site of the tumor and/or the type of the colectomy.

For rectal carcinomas, a total mesorectal excision should be used for tumors of the middle and lower third of the rectum, as part of either the low anterior or the abdominoperineal resection. For tumors of the upper third of the rectum, a tumor-specific mesorectal excision should be used with the mesorectum divided ideally no less than 5 cm below the lower margin of the tumor.

Those patients who are medically unfit for radical surgery, laparoscopic colectomy or mesorectal excision is strongly indicated in an elective setting. Numerous large multicenter, randomized, comparative trials have concluded that the laparoscopic approach has a much more uneventful postoperative course compared to that of the open approach. Patients after laparoscopic resection can also enroll to an enhanced recovery program ("fast-track" surgery), assuring that they will recover quicker, with less postoperative complications, fewer days of in-hospital stay, and subsequently less total health care cost.

The oncological outcome defined as *tumor-free resection margins* and the necessary number of retrieved lymph nodes are similar between the two approaches. Furthermore, local recurrence and disease-related survival are also comparable

Table 3.3 Stage grouping

Stage 0	Tis	N	M
Stage I	T1	0	0
Stage II	T2	N	M
Stage IIA	T3, T4	0	0
Stage IIB	T3	N	M
Stage IIC	T4a	0	0
Stage III		N	M
Stage IIIA	T1	N2a	M0
Stage IIIB	T1, T2	N2b	M0
	T2, T3	N2a	M0
	T3, T4a	N1	M0
Stage IIIC	T3, T4a	N2b	M0
	T4a	N2a	M0
	T4b	N1, N2	M0
Stage IV	Any T	Any N	M1
Stage IVA	Any T	Any N	M1a
Stage IVB	Any T	Any N	M1b
Stage IVC	Any T	Any N	M1c

between the two approaches. Long-term outcomes concerning morbidity are in favor of laparoscopic approach; incidence of obstructive ileus and incisional hernia is remarkably less after laparoscopy.

Patient's age should not be considered as a contraindication for minimal invasive colon surgery. Laparoscopic surgery can be also used for elder patients with poor performance status, as it offers all the benefits mentioned above. It was believed, though, that patients with poor performance status have higher rate of postoperative cardiac and respiratory complications as a result of the longer duration of surgery, pneumoperitoneum, and extreme Trendelenburg position, which are associated with laparoscopy. However, open surgery results in more surgical stress, which may lead to significant postoperative morbidity and mortality in patients with poor performance status. Nevertheless, laparoscopic surgery for colorectal carcinoma should be performed only by experienced surgeons, in high-volume centers. It was believed that the presence of locally advanced colorectal cancer ($\geq$T4) should be a contraindication for laparoscopic approach, as the tumor and the involved adjacent organs should be removed *en bloc*.[1] Multiple large clinical trials and meta-analyses have shown no significant difference in disease-free survival among patients operated laparoscopically and those operated conventionally. Tumor can be completely resected (R0) with both approaches, yet with open approach more lymph nodes can be retrieved. Theoretically, the extend of lymphadenectomy is considered a prognostic factor, but this has not yet been proven to affect the overall survival. According to the latest UICC recommendations, at least 12 lymph nodes must be retrieved; it has been shown that this threshold can be also achieved with laparoscopy. Nevertheless, locally advanced colorectal cancer requires conversion to laparotomy in almost 20% of the cases [22]. A conversion due to intraoperative difficulties is not correlated, however, with higher morbidity or mortality rate. Therefore, especially for T4a tumors, an exploratory laparoscopy should be initially performed and, depending on the intraoperative findings, a conversion to open surgery could follow. For T4b tumors, the choice of surgical approach is dependent on the nature of the multivisceral resection required to achieve negative margins. For example, duodenal involvement is an absolute contraindication for laparoscopic approach. Therefore, bad outcomes of laparoscopic treatment of T4b tumors are reported rarely, and no significant difference between the two operative approaches, in terms of survival, are observed.

For carcinomas of transverse colon, minimal invasive colectomy is contraindicated because of technical difficulties arising from the dissection of the middle colic vessels; other than this, the quality of the specimen is not optimal. Obesity and ASA score are also considered contraindication, as discussed earlier. Finally, laparoscopic procedures are not indicated in acutely perforated or obstructing colonic tumors, where an emergency explorative laparotomy is needed.

---

[1] *En bloc:* The resection of a bulky tumor without dissection. This method is used mainly for removing the primary lesion, the contiguous lymph nodes, and the in-between in certain cancers.

3.4   Conclusions

All in all, laparoscopic colorectal surgery emerges as a safe alternative to open surgery, with unquestionable advantages in terms of early postoperative morbidity and even mortality. Long-term outcomes of minimal invasive approach are comparable and, in many cases, superior to those of open surgery, while oncological outcomes of laparoscopy are encouraging. Still, for emergencies, or for complex surgical pathologies, the open approach remains the method of choice. Moreover, factors that are not strictly related to the technique, such as lack of operative time, available personnel, play an important role in deciding which approach to follow. Therefore, a proper preoperative selection of patients undergoing laparoscopy is essential. Large, intensive training programs are also required, for more surgeons to get familiar with minimal invasive techniques.

American Society of Anesthesiologists' Risk Classification (ASA) Status

ASA status	Definition	Examples
I	A normal healthy patient	Healthy, nonsmoking, no or minimal alcohol use
II	A patient with mild systemic disease	Mild diseases only without substantive functional limitations
		Examples include (but not limited to) current smoker, social alcohol drinker, pregnancy, obesity (30 < BMI < 40), mild lung disease
III	A patient with severe systemic disease	Substantive functional limitations; one or more moderate to severe diseases. Examples include (but not limited to) poorly controlled Diabetes mellitus, chronic obstructive pulmonary disease, morbid obesity (BMI $\geq$40), active hepatitis, alcohol dependence or abuse, implanted pacemaker, moderate reduction of ejection fraction
IV	A patient with severe systemic disease that is a constant threat to life	Examples include (but not limited to) ongoing cardiac ischemia or severe valve dysfunction, severe reduction of ejection fraction, sepsis, disseminated intravascular coagulation, acute respiratory distress syndrome, or renal failure not undergoing regularly scheduled dialysis
V	A moribund patient who is not expected to survive without the operation	Examples include (but not limited to) ruptured abdominal/ thoracic aneurysm, massive trauma, intracranial bleed with mass effect, ischemic bowel in the face of significant cardiac pathology or multiple organ/system dysfunction
VI	A declared brain-dead patient whose organs are being removed for donor purposes	

References

1. Jacobs M, Verdeja JC, et al. Minimally invasive colon resection (laparoscopic colectomy). Surg Laparosc Endosc. 1991;1:144–50.
2. Abraham NS, Young JM, Solomon MJ. Meta-analysis of short-term outcomes after laparoscopic resection for colorectal cancer. Br J Surg. 2004;91:1111–24.
3. Veldkamp R, Kuhry E, Hop WC, Jeekel J, Kazemier G, Bonjer HJ, et al. Laparoscopic surgery versus open surgery for colon cancer: short-term outcomes of a randomised trial. Lancet Oncol. 2005;6:477–84.
4. Bosker RJI, Van't Riet E, de Noo M, Vermaas M, Karsten TM, Pierie JP. Minimally invasive versus open approach for right-sided colectomy: a study in 12,006 patients from the Dutch surgical colorectal audit. Dig Surg. 2018;36(1):27–32. https://doi.org/10.1159/000486400.
5. Fugang W, Zhaopeng Y, Meng Z, Maomin S. Long-term outcomes of laparoscopy vs. open surgery for colorectal cancer in elderly patients: a meta-analysis. Mol Clin Oncol. 2017;7:771–6. https://doi.org/10.3892/mco.2017.1419.
6. Zeng WG, Zhou ZX, Hou HR, Liang JW, Zhou HT, Wang Z, Zhang XM, Hu JJ. Outcome of laparoscopic versus open resection for rectal cancer in elderly patients. J Surg Res. 2015;193:613–8.
7. Jiang JB, Jiang K, Wang JJ, Dai Y, Xie FB, Li XM. Short-term and long-term outcomes regarding laparoscopic versus open surgery for low rectal cancer: a systematic review and meta-analysis. Surg Laparosc Endosc Percutan Tech. 2015;25:286–96.
8. Niitsu H, Hinoi T, Kawaguchi Y, Ohdan H, Hasegawa H, Suzuka I, Fukunaga Y, Yamaguchi T, Endo S, Tagami S, Idani H, Ichihara T, Watanabe K, Watanabe M, Japan Society of Laparoscopic Colorectal Surgery. Laparoscopic surgery for colorectal cancer is safe and has survival outcomes similar to those of open surgery in elderly patients with a poor performance status: subanalysis of a large multicenter case-control study in Japan. J Gastroenterol. 2016;51:43–54. https://doi.org/10.1007/s00535-015-1083-y.
9. Alnasser M, Schneider EB, et al. National disparities in laparoscopic colorectal procedures for colon cancer. Surg Endosc. 2014;28:49–57.
10. Verzaro R, Mattia S, Rago T, Casella F, Ferroni A, Gianfreda V, Cofini V, Necozione S. Selection bias in colorectal surgery in a non-tertiary hospital: laparoscopic versus open surgery. J Laparoendosc Adv Surg Tech A. 2018;28:263–8. https://doi.org/10.1089/lap.2017.0174.
11. Marks JH, Kawun UB, Hamdan W, Marks G. Redefining contraindications to laparoscopic colorectal resection for high-risk patients. Surg Endosc. 2008;22:1899–904. https://doi.org/10.1007/s00464-008-9828-9; Epub 2008 Mar 18.
12. Bernell O, Lapidus A, Hellers G. Risk factors for surgery and postoperative recurrence in Crohn's disease. Ann Surg. 2000;231:38–45.
13. Schmidt CM, Talamini MA, Kaufman HS, Lilliemoe KD, Learn P, Bayless T. Laparoscopic surgery for Crohn's disease: reasons for conversion. Ann Surg. 2001;233:733–9.
14. Maggiori L, Panis Y. Laparoscopy in Crohn's disease. Best Pract Res Clin Gastroenterol. 2014;28:183–94. https://doi.org/10.1016/j.bpg.2013.11.004.
15. Bach SP, Mortensen NJ. Ileal pouch surgery for ulcerative colitis. World J Gastroenterol. 2007;28(13):3288–2300.
16. Marcello PW, Schoetz DJ, Roberts PL, Murray JJ, Coller JA, Rusin LC, Veidenheimer MC. Evolutionary changes in the pathologic diagnosis after the ileoanal pouch procedure. Dis Colon Rectum. 1997;40:263–9.
17. Ahmed Ali U, Keus F, Heikens JT, Bemelman WA, Berdah SV, Gooszen HG, van Laarhoven CJ. Open versus laparoscopic (assisted) ileo pouch anal anastomosis for ulcerative colitis and familial adenomatous polyposis. Cochrane Database Syst Rev. 2009;21:CD006267. https://doi.org/10.1002/14651858.CD006267.pub2.
18. Koh CE, Juszczyk K, Cooper MJ, Solomon MJ. Management of deeply infiltrating endometriosis involving the rectum. Dis Colon Rectum. 2012;55:925–31. https://doi.org/10.1097/DCR.0b013e31825f3092.

19. Sartelli M, Catena F, Ansaloni L, Coccolini F, Griffiths EA, Abu-Zidan FM, di Saverio S, Ulrych J, Kluger Y, Ben-Ishay O, Moore FA, Ivatury RR, Coimbra R, Peitzman AB, Leppaniemi A, Fraga GP, Maier RV, Chiara O, Kashuk J, Sakakushev B, Weber DG, Latifi R, Biffl W, Bala M, Karamarkovic A, Inaba K, Ordonez CA, Hecker A, Augustin G, Demetrashvili Z, Melo RB, Marwah S, Zachariah SK, Shelat VG, McFarlane M, Rems M, Gomes CA, Faro MP, Júnior GAP, Negoi I, Cui Y, Sato N, Vereczkei A, Bellanova G, Birindelli A, di Carlo I, Kok KY, Gachabayov M, Gkiokas G, Bouliaris K, Çolak E, Isik A, Rios-Cruz D, Soto R, Moore EE. WSES guidelines for the management of acute left sided colonic diverticulitis in the emergency setting. World J Emerg Surg. 2016;11:37. https://doi.org/10.1186/s13017-016-0095-0.
20. Bujanda L, Cosme A, Gil I, Arenas-Mirave JI. Malignant colorectal polyps. World J Gastroenterol. 2010;16:3103–11.
21. Brierley J, Gospodarowicz M, Wittekind C. TNM classification of malignant tumours, 8th ed. Willey Blackwell; 2017, ISBN: 978-1-119-26357-9.
22. Buunen M, Veldkamp R, Hop WC, Kuhry E, Jeekel J, Haglind E, et al. Survival after laparoscopic surgery versus open surgery for colon cancer: long-term outcome of a randomised clinical trial. Lancet Oncol. 2009;10:44–52.

Instruments

Ioannis Makris, Vasileios Papaziogas,
and Eugenia (Jenny) Matsiota

4.1   Introduction

Since the performance of the first laparoscopic colon procedure in 1991 [1], laparoscopic colorectal surgery has evolved to an advanced procedure for the surgical treatment of the whole spectrum of benign and malignant diseases of the colon and rectum. The initial concerns of possible adverse effects of laparoscopy on the oncological outcomes of patients with colorectal cancer were not justified. Many randomized trials showed no difference between the oncology results of laparoscopic colon surgery and the open surgical procedure [2–4]. The oncological outcomes (number of retrieved lymph nodes, R0 resections, survival rates, recurrence rates) were similar between the two surgical techniques.

This progress could not have been achieved without the significant evolution of the instrumentation of laparoscopic surgery and the whole setup of the operating room [5]. A major breakthrough was the development of instruments allowing both dissection and hemostasis (e.g., the ultrasonic or bipolar scissors), which led to the significant decrease of the duration of advanced laparoscopic procedures, as well as to the significant decrease of intraoperative blood loss. Furthermore, the evolution of the imaging equipment from simple three-chip cameras to ultra-, high-definition

I. Makris
Professor Emeritus (Retired), School of Medicine, Aristotle University of Thessaloniki,
Thessaloniki, Greece

V. Papaziogas
Director of 2nd Surgery Clinic of AUTH, Professor of Surgery AUTH, School of Medicine,
Aristotle University of Thessaloniki, Thessaloniki, Greece

University of Munich, Munich, Germany

E. (J.) Matsiota (✉)
Visiting Professor, Public Administration and Liberal Arts, Hankuk University of Foreign
Studies, Seoul, Republic of Korea

© The Editor(s) (if applicable) and The Author(s),
under exclusive license to Springer Nature Switzerland AG 2021
G. Kouraklis, E. (J.) Matsiota (eds.), *Laparoscopic Colon Surgery*,
https://doi.org/10.1007/978-3-030-56728-6_4

cameras of three-dimensional imaging analysis allowed for better perception of the operative field, leading to more precise and bloodless dissections.

The global market value of laparoscopic devices is expected to be \$12.3 billion by 2024 [6]. The main market players are B. Braun Melsungen AG, Boston Scientific Corp., CONMED Corporation, Ethicon Endo-Surgery, Inc., Intuitive Surgical, Inc., and Karl Storz GmbH & Co. KG [6]. These companies have developed and continue to develop technologically advanced instruments that make the surgical operation easier and safer. Nevertheless, extensive training is required for surgeons to acquaint themselves with new surgical instruments and use them efficiently. This chapter presents the instruments required for the performance of laparoscopic colectomy. Most of these instruments are used also in any laparoscopic procedure.

4.2   Patient's and Surgeon's Positioning

The correct positioning of the patient on the operating table is very important to facilitate safe exposure of the operative field and ergonomic placement of the laparoscopic instruments. For laparoscopic procedures, which do not necessitate intraoperative colonoscopy or access to the anus for circular stapling, the supine position is ideal (e.g., right hemicolectomy or ileocecal resection). In cases of low anterior rectum, resection, or abdominoperineal resection, surgeons prefer usually the modified lithotomy position. For right hemicolectomy, the surgeon and assistant usually stand at the left side of the patient, whereas for left colon resections, including low-rectum or abdominoperineal resections, the preferred position is at the right side of the patient [7] (Fig. 4.1). The positioning of the surgeon between the patient's legs

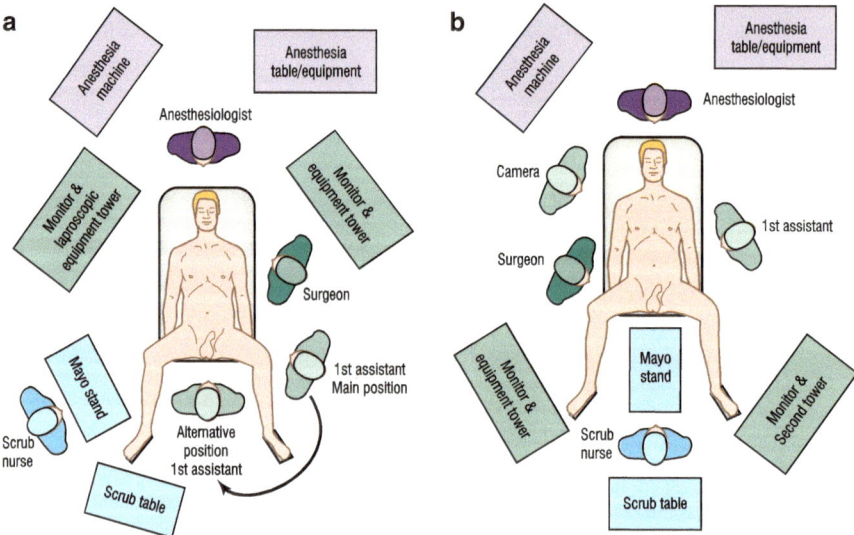

Fig. 4.1 Patient's and surgeon's positioning for right (**a**) and left (**b**) colonic resections. (Source: Tonia M. Young-Fadok (2006) [7]

allows easier approach for mobilization of the left colic flexure and detachment of the omentum from the transverse colon. The angle of the legs can be changed during the operation to allow freedom of movements for the surgeon. In cases of abdominoperineal resection, some surgeons prefer to complete the operation (after full mobilization of the rectum and exteriorization of the ostomy) in the prone position. The tacking of both arms parallel to the body of the patient is preferred to allow easy access of the surgeon to both sides of the patient. Due to the frequent, necessary changes of the position of the patient, the use of an electronically operated table is very useful. Deep Trendelenburg (head down) position combined with tilt to the right is essential for the retraction of the intestines from the pelvis in cases of low anterior resections. Tilt to the left is essential for removal of the small intestine from the operative field during a right hemicolectomy. Reverse Trendelenburg (head up) position is required for mobilization of the colonic flexures. The securing of the patient on the operating table during these intraoperative changes of position is essential to avoid nerve injuries.

4.3 Types of Instrument for Laparoscopic Colon Surgery

As in any laparoscopic procedure, the need is to create a working space within the abdomen, in order to perform the operation. For this purpose, the use of a controlled insufflation of CO_2 is mandatory. The controlled insufflator blows CO_2 into the abdominal cavity to create more workroom. The optical perception of the operative field is achieved utilizing an adequate light source, a laparoscope, and an image processing system, which projects the operative field on a monitor. The light is led from the light source through the laparoscope inside the operative field. The produced image is led through the laparoscope and processed digitally before presented on the monitor. The manipulation and dissection of the tissues are achieved with the use of a wide variety of laparoscopic instruments (atraumatic clamps, dissectors, scissors, etc.). Hemostasis is achieved with the use of ultrasonic or bipolar scissors. Greater vessels are ligated with the use of clips. The resection of the specimen and the restoration of the continuity of the gastrointestinal tract are performed with the use of stapling devices.

4.3.1 Insufflator

The preservation of an adequate operative workroom during the laparoscopic colorectal surgery is highly dependent on the use of a high-flow insufflator. A minimum of 10 l/min flow must be administered to establish and maintain pneumoperitoneum, even during the use of suction or smoke removal from the cannulas. Pneumatic insufflators cannot exceed 4 l/min flow. Therefore, the use of electronic insufflators is necessary because they can meet the required levels of insufflation. Electronic insufflators have digital displayed data concerning intra-abdominal pressure, delivered flow, and volume of consumed gas. The desired intra-abdominal pressure can be changed with the use of a pressure selector. The intraperitoneal pressure used for colorectal resections is approximately 14–15 mmHg.

To avoid sudden loss of vision, which impairs the surgical effectiveness and increases the operative time, new systems have been developed. The use of a heating and humidifying system of the gas is essential to avoid fogging of the lens of the laparoscope, which otherwise would require the repetitive removal of the scope from the abdomen; something that would increase operative time and the risk of injury and infection [8, 9]. The digital defogging (DD) system is a newly developed, advanced system that exports a dynamic, clear (defogged) image to the monitor [10]. Digital image processing involves algorithms that contribute to image processing in a digital way [10]. The result of DD is a clear image which is maintained throughout the laparoscopic colectomy. The clear vision helps the surgeon complete the operation sooner and promotes less surgical anxiety and less risk of injury and intraoperative complications.

4.3.2   Laparoscope

The laparoscope contains a bundle of optic fibers, which transfer the light from the light source to the operative filed, within the abdomen of the patient. In addition, the laparoscope contains a series of catoptric lenses, transferring the image from the operative field to the image processor, which is also connected to the laparoscope. Most surgeons prefer the use of an angled laparoscope, usually a 30° laparoscope. An angled scope offers better view but its use is more technically demanding and therefore the surgeon may need the support of an experienced assistant. The standard laparoscope is 10 mm in diameter; however, 5 mm laparoscopes may be used for single incision laparoscopic surgery (SILS) of the colon [8, 9].

4.3.3   Light Source

The standard light source is a 300-Watt xenon lamp. A *white balance*[1] procedure is recommended to optimize better transmission of the color quality [8, 9]. With *white balance,* the surgeon adjusts the intensity of the three basic colors (red, blue, and green) to accurately reproduce the white color. The camera is placed in front of a white surface (e.g., gaze) with the desired light intensity. The camera control unit is adjusted until it matches the color of the card on a *vectorscope.*[2] If any change in the light conditions occurs, the white balance procedure must be repeated. Adequate color quality allows better perception of the operative field, which enables more accurate movements and a more efficient surgical procedure.

---

[1] *White Balance* is a term used in digital photography. It is the adjustment of colors to make the image look more natural.

[2] *Vectorscope* is a special type of oscilloscope that is used to measure the color information of a video image.

4.3.4   Camera

Older generation laparoscopic 2D cameras used 1–3 silicon charge coupled devices (CCD) achieving a resolution of approximately 700–800 lines per inch. The use of high definition (HD) technology significantly increased the quality of the produced images (720 × 1280 pixels). Furthermore, 4 K (4096 × 2180 pixels) and Ultra HD resolution (UHD, 3840 × 2160 pixels) are available, which means four times more image information than Full HD (Olympus, Visera 4 K, UHD) (Fig. 4.2). The result of ultra-high-resolution images is that the size of the picture displayed on the monitor can be enlarged without compromising its quality. Thus, even fine anatomical structures can be identified and dissected, allowing a safe and quick dissection. A magnified visualization function allows the use of the laparoscope at a longer distance from the operating field, having the same picture quality, and thus avoiding collisions or "sword-fighting" with other laparoscopic instruments entered in the abdomen.

The three-dimensional (3D) technology has evolved in the last years mainly through robotic surgery, but has also been used in conventional laparoscopic surgery. 3D stereoscopic image is offering a better understanding of the depth of the abdomen; something that has been compromised with the conventional 2D image processing, which was missing the depth perception [8, 9, 11–13].

4.3.5   Monitor

The use of a high-resolution monitor is essential to fully exploit the advantages provided by the advanced technology of image processing. To utilize the full benefit of HD imaging and maximize performance, the monitor resolution must be properly

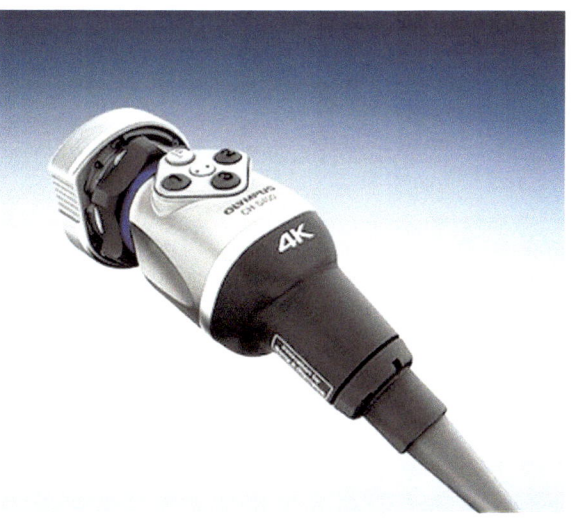

Fig. 4.2 4 K system for UHD viewing (Visera 4 K, Olympus)

matched to the resolution of the camera head [8, 11]. If the resolution of the monitor is lower than the resolution of the camera head, the result would be lower image quality displayed on the monitor. On the other hand, increase in the resolution of the monitor would also compromise image quality. The resolution between the camera head and the monitor has to be the same to achieve optimum image results.

4.3.6 Recording Devices

Digital documentation of laparoscopic procedures has been an important technological advancement helping surgeons to perform self-assessment and identify errors that may have caused intra or postoperative complications. Therefore, digital documentation ultimately contributes to surgical skills' improvement. Most recording systems used today are able to store the digital archive of the procedure in the hard disk of a connected computed. These files can be further processed to be stored or presented for scientific and other purposes [8, 9, 11, 12]. Prerecorded laparoscopic operations are widely used as a method of teaching new surgeons the laparoscopic techniques. Laparoscopic videos can be watched freely in the web. These videos provide, not only to the surgeons but also to the patients, valuable information about the laparoscopic procedures.

4.3.7 Entry Methods and Instrumentation

Laparoscopy is a blind procedure. Therefore, it constitutes a significant challenge for the surgeon who performs laparoscopic surgery to access the abdomen in a safe way, without causing any injuries. The main complications associated with entering the abdomen and maintaining pneumoperitoneum are subcutaneous emphysema, bleeding, gastrointestinal tract perforation, and injury of the vessels [14]. The number of injuries in laparoscopy is rare, (2 in 10,000 procedures), but these injuries have fatal results or serious complications. It is of critical importance to ensure safe entry to the abdomen. Three are the entry techniques:

- (1) the *Verres Needle* technique, (2) the *Hasson* technique, and (3) the *Direct Trocar* Insertion technique.

4.3.7.1 The Veress Needle Technique
The two most commonly used methods of entering the abdominal area are the closed technique (also known as the *Veress* needle technique and the open technique (also known as the *Hasson* technique). A third technique, mainly used by gynecologists, is the direct trocar insertion technique [14]. The Veress needles or, similar to the *Veress needles*, the disposable needles named *Auto Suture Surgineedle*[3]

---

[3] Trademark of the United States Surgical Corporation.

come in two lengths 120 mm and 150 mm and have an external diameter of 2 mm [15, 16]. Surgeons use them to enter the pneumoperitoneum in the virgin abdomen [16]. The *Veress* needle is the oldest entry method that Dr. Janos *Veress* developed in 1938, a Hungarian internist [15]. The main criticism about the use of this needle is that it compromises insufflation because it allows only slow insufflation rates [14] with life-threatening complications. The two most important aspects a surgeon should consider when entering the abdomen with the *Veress* needle are 1) to avoid excessive insertion that can injure big vessels and 2) to insert the needle up to that point as to avoid extraperitoneal insufflation [15]. The angle of insertion in nonobese patients should be 45° [17]. After insertion, the surgeon should test if the needle is inserted correctly. Different methods and assisting technologies exist to ensure safe insertion of the needle. Nevertheless, errors occur with detrimental consequences for the patient. Therefore, it is of critical importance to adequately train surgeons to perform laparoscopic colectomy in a safe and efficient way. More information about training can be read in Chap. 8 of this book.

4.3.7.2 The Hasson Technique
Another entry technique is the *Hasson* technique which Dr. Hasson introduced in 1971 [15]. The Hasson technique is considered an open technique and requires a small incision of 1–2 cm long of the lower edge of the umbilical fossa [17]. Surgeons prefer this technique with high-risk patients, to avoid visceral injury, bowel injury from the puncture, gas embolism, and preperitoneal insufflation [15]. The main criticism about this technique is that it takes time, has higher degree of difficulty, especially with obese patients, and is hard to keep the pneumoperitoneum [15, 17]. As in the case of the *Verres* needle, similarly with the Hasson technique, experience built through practice and training is critical to avoid errors and complications, especially in the case of highly demanding surgical procedures like the laparoscopic colectomy.

4.3.7.3 The Direct Trocar Insertion Technique
A third method of entering the peritoneum is the *direct trocar insertion* technique, which was established by Dr. Dingfelder in 1978 [14]. With this technique, the surgeon inserts the trocar without creating pneumoperitoneum. The patient is placed in a supine position. The surgeons create a wide incision to allow the entrance of the trocar, lift the abdominal wall manually by pulling two towel clips placed on either side of the umbilicus to insert the trocar in an angle of 90° [17].

The *Veress* needle technique is the oldest but is not considered the safest. An increasing number of studies support that the *Hasson* technique (open method) and the *direct trocar insertion* technique are the safest entry methods with less complications for their patients compared to the *Veress* technique [14, 15, 17]. Even though in the case of direct or open access, extensive training is required for the surgeon to perform successfully the first step in any laparoscopic surgery, which is the insertion of the trocar in the abdominal area.

Trocars

The most common direct-puncture trocars surgeons use in most second- and third-generation laparoscopic procedures have diameters of around 10 mm, 12 mm, and 15 mm [16]. Long versions of trocars of these diameters exist but they are rarely used, mainly in cases of obese patients, although the standard sizes usually work with obese patients too. In the case surgeons follow the *Hasson* technique to enter the peritoneum, they use a blunt trocar, which does not require previous pneumoperitoneum. The number and type of trocars used for laparoscopic colorectal surgery depend on the preferences of the surgeon. In both the *Veress needle* technique and the *Hasson* technique, the site of entrance is usually the umbilical region.

Surgeons use the *stationary or traction trocars* to insert instruments for retraction or traction purposes laparoscopically. The *working trocar* is used to allow surgeons to pass instruments for dissection, clipping, cutting, stapling, or suturing. Finally, the *scope trocar* is used to enter the laparoscope [16]. The introduction of an endostapler necessitates the use of at least one 12 mm trocar. The site of insertion of this trocar is chosen so that it can provide easy access to the part of the colon to be resected. For left colonic resections, the site of the 12 mm trocar is usually in the right iliac fossa.

Trocars should be placed distant from each other to avoid jamming and in the correct position to make the laparoscopic procedure easier and faster. Also, the minimum possible diameter should be chosen to avoid trauma. If reusable metallic trocars are used, care should be taken to avoid any direct or indirect contact to the electrocautery to avoid electrothermal injuries [8, 9, 18]. The operating room team should have an extensive training to possess a thorough understanding of the fundamentals of electrosurgery to ensure patient safety.

4.3.7.4 Grasping and Dissecting Instruments

Manipulating the tissue using laparoscopic *forceps* and *graspers* is harder from using the hand. In the beginning, graspers were long and rigid without much of haptic feedback. As a result, it was hard for the surgeon to control the force he or she was applying on the tissue. In cases extensive force was applied damaging the tissue or loose force was applied and the tissue was slipping from the grasper. According to clinical studies, a colectomy could last from 24 to 119 minutes and the surgeon had to clamp the colon many times with a success rate of grasping of 63% [19]. Throughout the years, technology progressed and the design of graspers has become friendlier to the surgeons' movements, offering better haptic feedback, and safer for the patients. Grasping instruments should allow for gentle holding of the colon minimizing the risk of serosal damage or hemorrhage. The use of atraumatic graspers, such as Babcock clamps (5 or 10 mm), is important to avoid inadvertent injury. Nevertheless, no matter how atraumatic a grasper can be, the surgeon needs to be very cautious and avoid grasping the mesocolon because it is more fragile than the colon and therefore prone to hemorrhage [8, 9].

Dissection can be achieved with the use of *hooks, scissors,* or *dissecting clamps.* These instruments can be introduced through 5 mm or 5–10 (5–12) mm trocars.

Dissecting and grasping instruments can be connected to monopolar electrocautery to be used simultaneously for hemostasis.

Endoscopic *needle holders* are used when the application of sutures is necessary a) for the closure of the intestine after application of the endostapler, b) for covering the endostapler line with an additional suture line, and c) for reaching the mesentery after the anastomosis. Linear as well as curved needle holders are available in various forms according to the preferences and the experience of the surgeon [8, 9]. Laparoscopic colectomy is a very demanding surgery and the manipulation of instruments is a hard task even for experienced surgeons. To enhance skill advancement and patient safety, simulation training systems have been developed to simulate colectomy with patient specific data. These simulation systems utilize 3D computer-aided design data to reconstruct laparoscopic instruments to simulate surgical manipulations with the use of PHANTOM[4] devices [21]. More about contemporary methods of training will be discussed in the chapter of education and best practices (Chap. 8 of this book).

4.3.8 Endoscopic Devices for Anastomosis

Anastomosis is a crucial step in laparoscopic colectomy because it determines early and late postoperative complications. The most common tools for anastomosis, for years, have been sutures and staplers. There is controversy among surgeons about which of the two, sutures or staples, are better for colorectal anastomosis but no consensus has been reached, with most surgeons arguing that it is mostly a matter of personal preference and availability. The main disadvantage of vascular endostaplers is that they usually need a dissection of the vessel of at least 1–2 cm to pass behind it. They are quick and safe but significantly expensive [8, 9]. Also, staplers have a relatively high incidence rate of strictures and intraoperative accidents [22]. The use of surgical sutures causes inflammatory reaction, either these are absorbable or are nonabsorbable [22]. Silk sutures may cause a persisting for weeks inflammatory reaction. Polypropylene and polyglycolic sutures have a milder reaction.

Connecting two parts of the intestine after dissection has been studied since the nineteenth century. The concept of compression anastomosis was introduced by Dr. Denan in 1826 [22]. In 1892, Dr. Murphy developed a simple metallic button, The *Murphy Button*, which has two hollow steel cylinders. This was considered the first sutureless anastomosis [22]. Since then, many devices have been developed that helped the technique of anastomosis. In recent years, the introduction of super-elastic clips and rings have contributed much the results of anastomosis [23]. There are four main types of compression anastomosis devices: (1) AKA-2, (2) Valtrac BAR, (3) compression anastomotic clip, and (4) endoluminal compression anastomotic ring.

---

[4] PHANTOM are devices that allow the surgeon to touch objects in a virtual environment having a haptic feedback. The first PHANTOM was developed by Thomas Massie, an American engineer and politician [20].

Fig. 4.3 AKA-2 ring
(INNOMEDICUS)

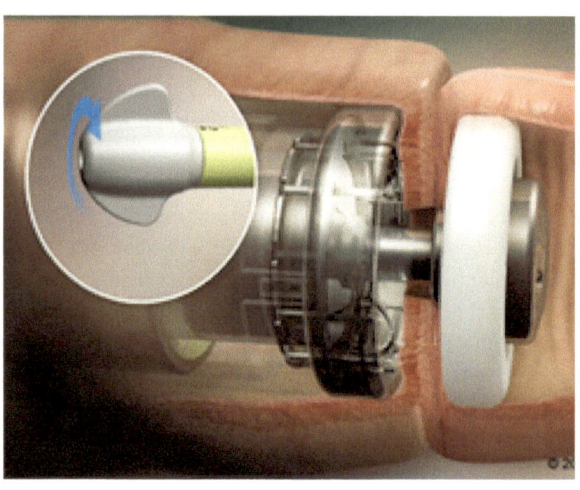

4.3.8.1 AKA-2

AKA-2 is a device used for transanal compression anastomosis. It has two rings, a base ring and a plastic ring (Fig. 4.3). The base ring is attached to the plastic ring (proximal ring) through metal pins and springs [22]. It was created in 1984 by a group of Russian scientists [24]. AKA-2 rings are applied with a transanal applicator. The circular blades cut the central cuff of the bowel and the pins apply compression on the inverted bowel edges. The components of AKA-2 are dislodged from the anastomosis after a period of 4–6 days and are excreted with feces [22]. The main advantage of AKA-2 device is that it helps the surgeon create a good lumen size to allow stool passage. Findings of a study that included 442 consecutive patients showed that the device is safe, demonstrating good healing results after compression [25].

4.3.8.2 Valtrac BAR

The Valtrac BAR ring (Fig. 4.4) is a development of the AKA-2 device. Hardy and colleagues invented a biofragmentable anastomosis ring (BAR; Valtrac) in 1987 [26]. It was a new technique in gastrointestinal surgery that facilitated the anastomosis process. The Valtrac BAR is an anastomotic ring that has two components which interlock on a central frame; one component is of absorbable polyglycolic acid (87.5%) and the other is of barium sulfate (12.5%) [22] (Fig. 4.3). Around this central frame, the tissue ends are connected by purse string sutures for anastomosis [27]. The BAR ring holds the parts of the intestine together. This device became popular in the 1990s. According to several studies, surgeons consider Valtrac BAR as easy or as difficult as suture or stapled anastomosis [22]. Others consider it a cumbersome process and the device bulky and inconvenient.

The ring devices hold together the ends of the intestine because of applied compression and are considered therefore responsible for recorded cases of necrosis [24]. Another concern with the device is that some surgeons apply high pressure and as a result the device may shatter to pieces. Rings with better shape and memory have been developed, made from nickel titanium (nitinol), that are safer and

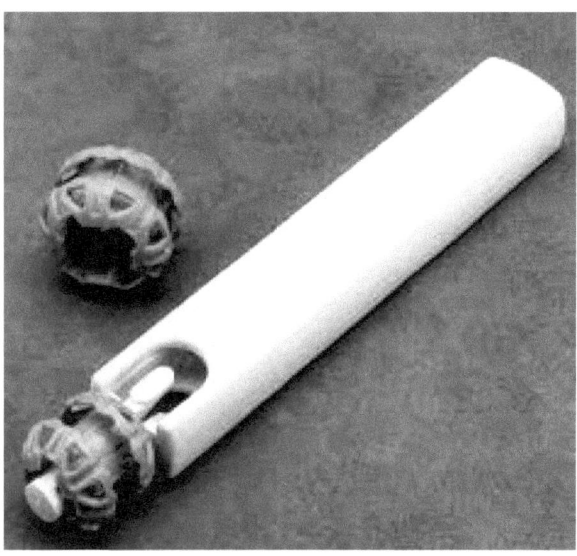

Fig. 4.4 Valtrac BAR (Stewart & Seim, et al.)

more effective. Nevertheless, the quality of perioperative anastomosis and the effect on the healing process have not been proven or monitored. Some of the main limitations of the Valtrac BAR are (1) mucosal tears, (2) device-locking failure, and (3) cases of postoperative and overcompressed lumen that constraints feces passage [22].

4.3.8.3 Compression Anastomotic Clips (CAC)

There is consensus among many studies that compression anastomotic clips are safe and effective with minimal inflammatory response and foreign body reaction, forming a very small scar tissue at the anastomotic line. The most common compression anastomotic clip is a temperature sensitive clip of a shape memory alloy (SMA) of nickel and titanium (Nitinol). Nitinol is formatted under high temperatures and it keeps its shape in a room temperature. Nitinol loses its rigidity and becomes more flexible when put in a temperature below zero Celsius [22]. This metal alloy is used extensively in the medical practice as for fixation of bone fractures or for vascular prosthesis.

The SMA device used for colon or bowel anastomosis comes in a form of a clip (compression anastomotic clip—CAC) or in a form of a ring (compression anastomotic ring—CAR). CAR will be presented in the next section under endoluminal compression anastomotic ring. The Nitinol CAC has a double ring which at zero Celsius stays open and is flexible. When the ring gets the body temperature, it closes holding the bowel tissue under compression (Fig. 4.5). The rings' internal diameter is 8 mm and is pierced with a blade applicator of 5 mm to restore bowel function after surgery. CAC, 1 week after surgery, detaches from the healthy tissue and is expelled from the body with feces.

The findings of a study having enrolled 63 patients with indications for enterocolic surgery indicate that CAC is a safe and effective device and an efficacious alternative to suturing or stapling anastomosis techniques [29]. A more recent retrospective study, published in 2016 that included 14 patients suffering from

Fig. 4.5 CAC device (Quintín Héctor González, et al. [28])

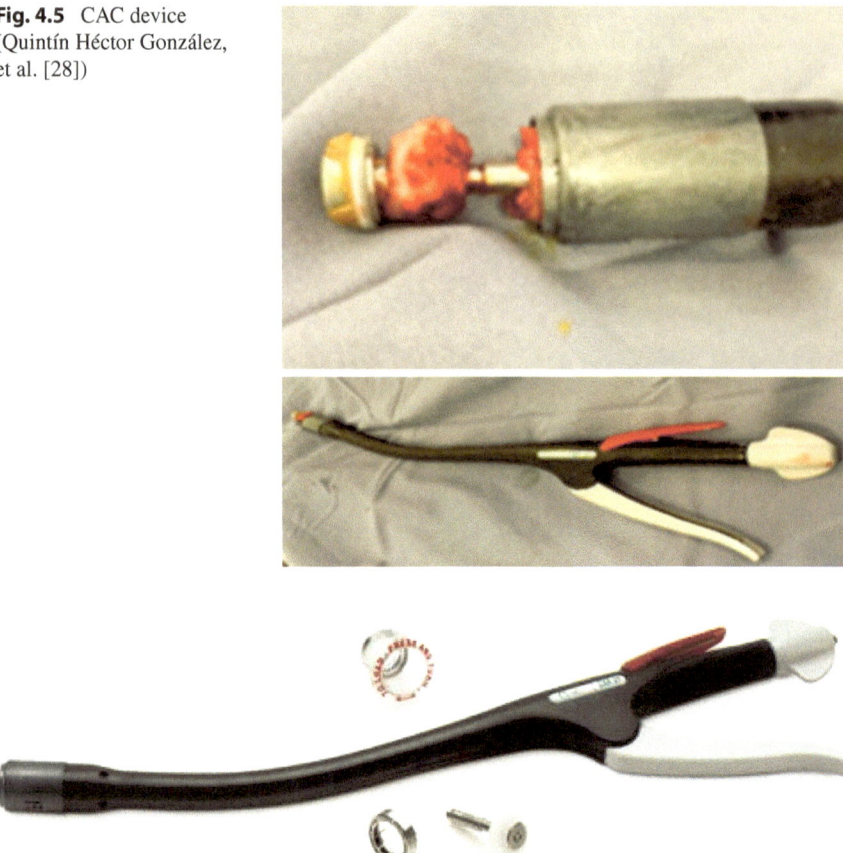

Fig. 4.6 Compression anastomotic ring (CAR) (Lee et al., 2011—[30])

complicated diverticular disease Hinchey II–III, showed that CAC is a good and safe alternative to sutures for colorectal anastomosis [28].

The main concern for colorectal surgeons is the complications following anastomosis like dehiscence, which may cause sepsis, fistula, stenosis, and, in some cases, may bring death. CAC seems to be a safe device that can help surgeons perform an effective anastomosis. The main disadvantage of the device is that it requires suture closure of the incision in the bowel wall through which the device is entered [22].

4.3.8.4 Endoluminal Compression Anastomotic Ring

The endoluminal compression anastomotic ring (CAR) (Fig. 4.6) has two separate synthetic rings that are attached to the body of the instrument in a very similar way like a circular stapler. One ring is mounted to the proximal bowel end and the instrument carrying the other ring is inserted through the anus to achieve rectal anastomosis. After the engagement, the rings are held together with Nitinol springs that apply the desired pressure. The surgeon uses a circular knife to resect the access tissue. After 7–10 days of surgery, the device is expelled naturally together with the necrosis [22].

A study of left-sided colonic resection, where CAR was used, showed that it was safe and efficacious alternative to suturing or stapling anastomosis [30]. An important study of 1180 patients who had end-to-end colorectal anastomosis with CAR proved the device to be safe and effective [31].

Colorectal anastomosis remains a demanding technique, associated with the most common complications of laparoscopic colectomy. Although many devices have been developed, nevertheless a standard, favorite procedure has not yet prevailed. Compression anastomosis has been around for years but still surgeons are reluctant to adhere to it despite of most studies showing that the technique is safe and efficacious, ensuring good results and patient safety. Ho and Tawfik in their work about *Techniques of colorectal anastomosis* [22] have summarized the existing techniques and devices and offer a detailed and comprehensive information about what is available. They have formatted a table that summarizes the characteristics of the four main compression devices. For the readers who desire a more detailed information about colorectal anastomosis techniques, the publication of Ho and Tawfik is highly recommended.

4.3.9 Devices for Vessel Ligation

Several types of clipping devices can be used for the ligation of large vessels like the inferior mesenteric artery in anterior rectum resection or the ileocolic artery in the right hemicolectomy. In the beginning, surgeons were using sutures, stapling devices, and titanium and polymer clips to manage hemostasis [32].

4.3.9.1 Titanium Clips

Large titanium clips may withstand high bursting pressure. Their advantage is that they can be applied even if the vessel is not fully dissected. This can be useful in case the vessel, the surgeon wants to ligate, is bleeding. Their main disadvantage is that they carry a risk of dislodgement lacking a locking mechanism. Therefore, it is advisable that at least three clips are applied proximally before cutting the vessel. Another disadvantage of large titanium clips is that they can transport electrical energy, thus surgeons should avoid contact of the colon with the coagulating device throughout the operation. Finally, because they act as foreign bodies within the abdominal cavity, they can cause adhesion formation.

Titanium clips may be applied either with a single-use clip applicator, which allows for immediate recharging and reapplication of up to 20 clips, or with a multiple-use clip applicator, which is charged by the nurse after each clip application.

4.3.9.2 Polymer Clips

Polymer clips with locking mechanism (hem-o-lok clips) allow safer ligation of the vessels, with minimal risk of dislodgement because of the existing locking

Fig. 4.7 Hem-o-lok clip
(Weck® Hem-o-lok®,
Teleflex)

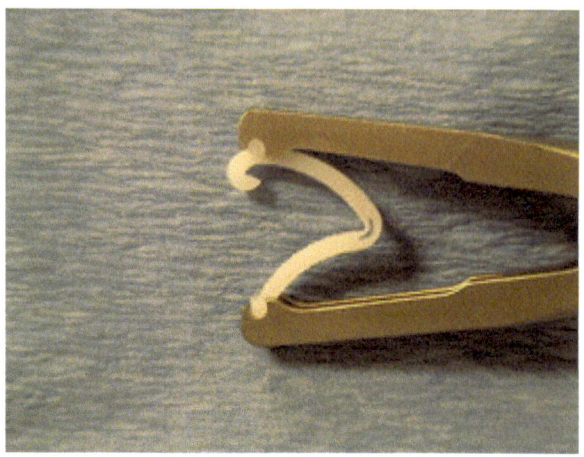

mechanism (Fig. 4.7). In addition, the locking mechanism provides a tactile feedback before closing. However, their application may be difficult or even impossible if the vessel is not fully dissected because their locking mechanism cannot close when tissue is around the vessel. Once placed, their removal is difficult. Plastic, polymer clips are applied either with single-use, immediately recharging, or with multiple-use clip applicators.

4.3.9.3 Energy Sources

In laparoscopic, as in open surgery, surgeons achieve dissection of the anatomical planes with a combination of coagulation and cutting techniques. These are the two main therapeutic applications of electrosurgery. Perfect hemostasis is essential for the determination and preservation of the exact dissection plane during advanced laparoscopic procedures such as colorectal resections. Even minor hemorrhage or oozing may compromise the quality of the laparoscopic view. Excess bleeding may lead the surgeon to convert to open surgery. Hemostasis with the use of local pressure, suction, or clip application may be even more technically demanding for the surgeon thus increasing the duration of the procedure and the risk of conversion or inadvertent injury [11].

Three main energy sources are used in laparoscopic surgery: (a) monopolar diathermy, (b) bipolar diathermy, and (c) ultrasonic [33–37].

Monopolar Electrosurgery

Monopolar electrosurgery is widely used in laparoscopic surgery because it is inexpensive and quick. It can be used with conventional laparoscopic instruments such as hooks, dissectors, clamps, shears, scissors, and spatulas. Monopolar electro current passes through tissues with the use of two electrodes at the distal tip of the instrument [32]. With monopolar electrosurgery, electrical currency is transferred from the generator to the active electrode, to the instrument, and to the tissue where electrosurgery is applied [38]. The use of monopolar instruments allows the surgeon to combine dissection with hemostasis.

However, three main disadvantages tend to minimize the use of monopolar diathermy as the sole energy source in advanced colorectal laparoscopic surgery. The first disadvantage is that its hemostatic effect cannot cover larger vessels (>2–3 mm) as bipolar or ultrasonic devices do, thus necessitating the use of clips.

Second, the use of monopolar diathermy produces significant amount of smoke compared to the other two energy sources, thus compromising the operative field and necessitating repeated desufflation of the intraperitoneal air through one of the cannulas. If the "contaminated" air in the operating room, especially during lengthy operative procedures, has negative effects on the health of the medical and nursing team remains unknown. The use of aspiration combined with rapidly recirculating gas insufflators may reduce the need for air desufflation. However, the extra time, the use of an additional instrument, and the associated cost are an issue. Argon beam is considered a sophisticated high-frequency electrosurgery in which Argon gas is ionized and used to form a current between the Argon plasma arc and the tissue. This technique reduces smoke because of the reduced carbonization [38]. Nevertheless, the effectiveness of the Argon beam is disputable especially on bowel and bladder electrosurgery [38].

The third disadvantage of monopolar energy is that the risk of inadvertent thermal injury is considerable. Inadequate insulation of the instrument shaft is the main reason for thermal injuries after contact of the poorly insulated instrument with tissues such as the bowel or the vessels. Another reason of thermal injuries with monopolar electrosurgery is the coupling effect among instruments [33–35]. Direct coupling can happen after accidental direct contact of the instrument with the tissue, or because of the formation of an electrical arc between a metal instrument or object and the active electrode [32]. Capacitive coupling may take place when electrical current is transferred from the active electrode to adjacent materials through the intact insulation although there is no direct contact. The last phenomenon is mostly evident with longer instruments, narrow trocars, thinner insulation, and high voltages [32].

Surgeons should be extremely careful when using monopolar energy with patients having pacemakers or implantable cardiac defibrillators because it may reset the pacemaker device or cause wrong sensing [38]. In such patients, a cardiologist is strongly recommended to be present during surgery. Bipolar or ultrasonic energies are preferable solutions for patients with pacemakers because the energy does not go through the human body [38].

Bipolar Electrosurgery

The bipolar electrosurgery has an active and a return electrode combined in a single electrosurgical instrument with two small poles [32, 38]. The surgical instrument is usually in the form of forceps [38]. The active and return electrodes form a closed electrical circuit. The electrical circuit is not formed between the active electrode and the ground (through the grounding pad) as in monopolar diathermy. Therefore, the main advantage of bipolar against monopolar diathermy is the reduction of thermal spread and consequently the reduced risk of thermal injury of adjacent organs. Furthermore, due to the proximity of the electrodes, the power required to induce the same hemostatic effect is significantly smaller than in monopolar diathermy. Lower voltage limits the risks of surrounding tissue damage and capacitive coupling.

The most classical bipolar instrument is the Kleppinger forceps (Fig. 4.8). The bipolar devices available today use a combination of both physical pressure and electrical energy to create vessel fusion. Thus, vessels up to 7 mm can be safely ligated providing a sealing withstanding at least the threefold of the normal systolic blood pressure. Advanced bipolar instruments combine bipolar diathermy and ultrasonic technology offering better hemostasis and increased efficiency [32].

The main disadvantage of bipolar devices is that the surgeon has to cut the fused tissue after making a second maneuver. However, bipolar devices offer a tissue-response feedback mechanism, which is able to calculate the exact amount of energy necessary for the sealing of the grasped tissue. After completion of the sealing process, which varies in time depending on the thickness of the grasped tissue (2–10 s), an audible tone is produced. At that time, the cutting mechanism can be activated and the sealed tissue cut. It is important to note that the sealing procedure can be repeated more than once in order to achieve better hemostasis.

Bipolar energy is available both as 5 mm and 10 mm instruments as well as in different shapes (e.g., Maryland clamps or dolphin clamps) allowing better dissection of the tissue (Fig. 4.9). The most representative vessel sealing devices are LigaSure (Valleylab, Boulder, CO), EnSeal (SurgRx, Inc. Palo Alto, CA), Caiman (Aragon, Palo Alto, CA), and the Gyrus [32]. Doctors Camran Nezhat, Michael Lewis, and Louise King at their work *Laparoscopic Vessel Sealing Devices* [32]

Fig. 4.8 Kleppinger forceps

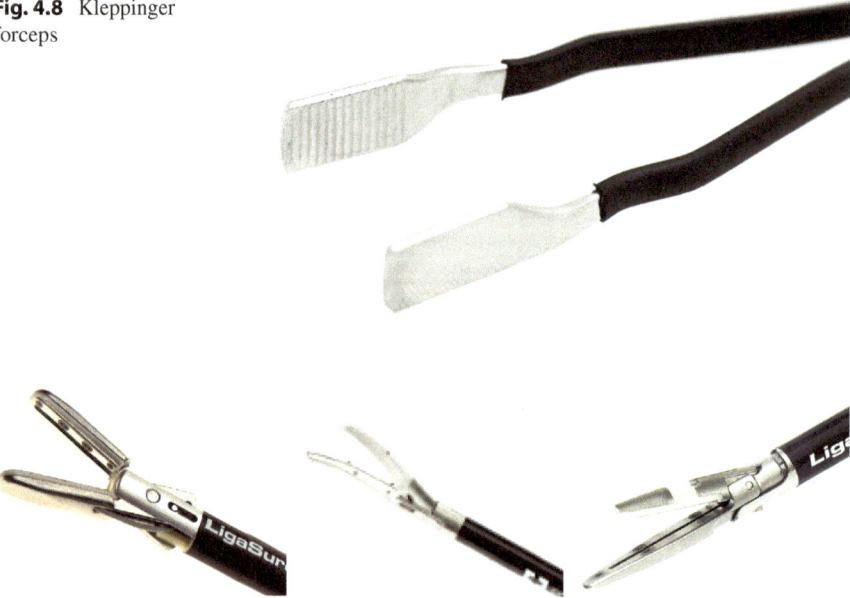

Fig. 4.9 Bipolar vessel sealing devises—LigaSure A. 10 mm (Atlas), 5 mm (Maryland), 5 mm (Dolphin)

explain the main characteristics of each of the aforementioned devices; part of their work will be presented below as a useful reference to the reader.

- *EnSeal* is a tissue sealing system that employs bipolar energy; there is an electrode in the plastic jaws of the instrument that concentrates energy on the tissue. This system utilizes a temperature sensitive matrix that aims to improve efficacy.
- *LigaSure* through its jaws delivers pressure as well as high current, low voltage energy on the tissue. The systems have the capability to monitor the energy expended while the collagen and the elastin within the vessel walls are denatured.
- *Caiman* is similar to LigaSure. The main advantage versus LigaSure is that it achieves less thermal spread and less operative time is required because of the bigger jaws with sealing length of 50 mm that it has.
- *Gyrus* uses plasma kinetic technology to deliver high current, low voltage energy. It is associated with lower thermal spread because of a series of rapid pulses that enhance cooling during coagulation.

Ultrasonic Energy

Ultrasonic energy uses the heating effect produced by vibrations (approximately 55,000 Hz) between the blades of the instrument. Ultrasonic systems include an ultrasonic generator, which converts electrical energy to ultrasonic frequency mechanical energy, and a hand instrument. The hand instrument consists of two jaws (blades): one passive and one active (oscillating blade). The heat denatures protein to form coagula. Therefore, the coagulating or cutting effect is achieved without any electricity flowing through the patient. In that respect it seems to be safer than electrocautery. However, the surgeon should keep in mind that the active blade can develop significant amount of thermal energy, thus the prolonged contact to the viscera or its use as a grasping forceps immediately after its use as an active blade should be avoided. Another advantage of ultrasonic energy is the minimal smoke compared to electrocautery. Ultrasonic dissectors are available only as 5 mm sized instruments. Three types of ultrasonic systems are available in the market: UltraCision harmonic scalpel (Ethicon Endo-Surgery, Cincinnati, OH), SonoSurg (Olympus), and AutoSonix (USSC, Tyco Healthcare) (Fig. 4.10).

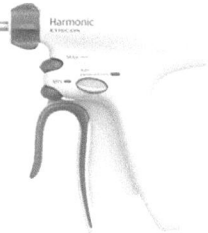

Fig. 4.10 Ultrasonic 5 mm scissors (HARMONIC ACE, Ethicon Endo-Surgery)

Fig. 4.11 Combination of ultrasonic and electrical energy (THUNDERBEAT, Olympus). (Source: http:// medical.olympusamerica. com/ products/ thunderbeat-0)

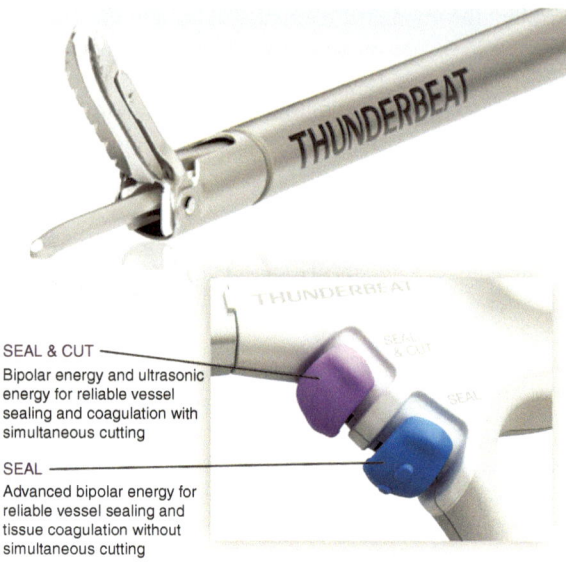

SEAL & CUT
Bipolar energy and ultrasonic energy for reliable vessel sealing and coagulation with simultaneous cutting

SEAL
Advanced bipolar energy for reliable vessel sealing and tissue coagulation without simultaneous cutting

Recently, a combination of ultrasonic and advanced bipolar energy was developed (THUNDERBEAT, Olympus). The new instrument allows the surgeon to perform two actions: seal (bipolar), and seal and cut (combined bipolar and ultrasonic energy) (Fig. 4.11) [33–37].

Radiofrequency Energy

Electrothermal bipolar vessel sealing as well as ultrasound energy are the latest advancements in technology that serve as a solution to the problems identified with monopolar and bipolar energies. The first device available for sealing vessels using radiofrequency (RF) energy was the TissueLink (TissueLink Medical, Inc., Dover, New Hampshire). In 2008, the company was renamed to Salient Medical Technologies until Medtronic acquired them in 2011. Radiofrequency energy is applied through a low-volume saline drip. The tip of the instrument cools and becomes a "wet electrode" sealing soft tissue without char or smoke [38]. The most advanced radiofrequency bipolar instrument is the Aquamantys Bipolar RF Sealers of Medtronic (Fig. 4.12).

The use of ultrasonic and radiofrequency energy sources is the latest energy sources used in laparoscopic colectomy aiming. These technologies aim to decrease operative time and smoke issues in the operating room that are usually the case with monopolar and bipolar energy sources. A meta-analysis in laparoscopic colectomy surgical procedures compared the effectiveness of ultrasonic with electrothermal bipolar energy sources indicating that the second is associated with lesser time in the operating room and less blood loss than the first [39]. Nevertheless, this meta-analysis serves as an indication and further studies would be required to offer more reliable evidence. It seems, though, that ultrasonic and radiofrequency energy use are the evolution of monopolar and bipolar electrosurgery in laparoscopic colectomy.

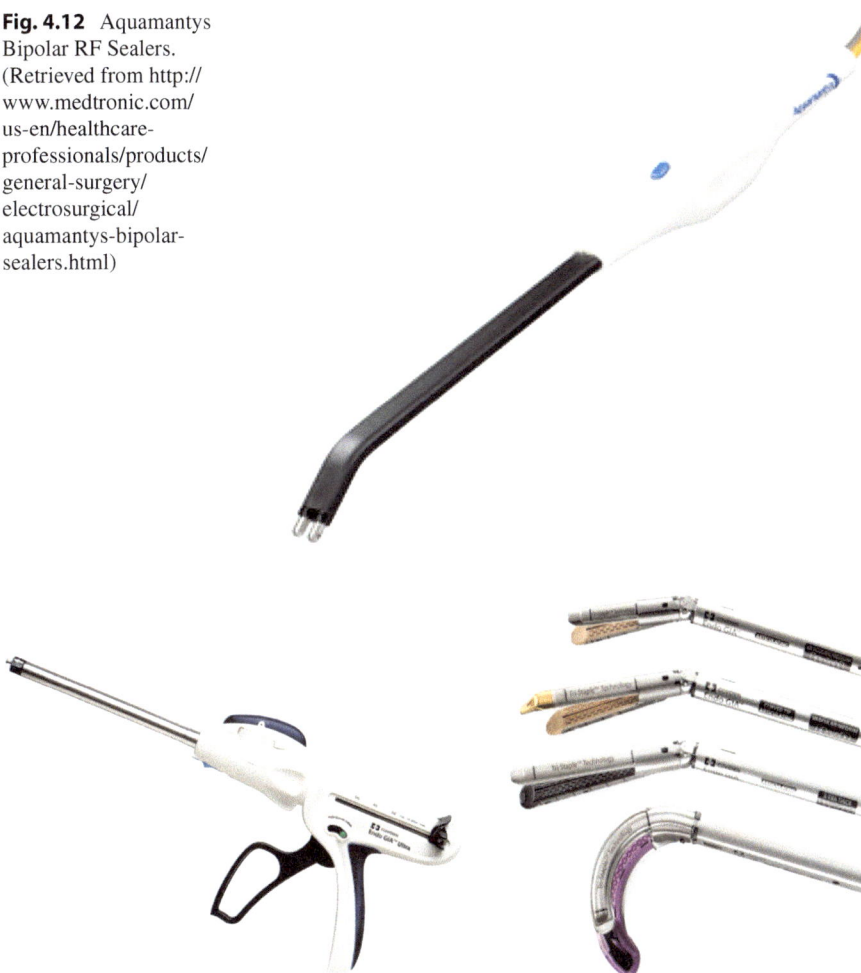

Fig. 4.12 Aquamantys Bipolar RF Sealers. (Retrieved from http://www.medtronic.com/us-en/healthcare-professionals/products/general-surgery/electrosurgical/aquamantys-bipolar-sealers.html)

Fig. 4.13 Endo GIA™ Ultra Universal Stapler. Covidien

4.3.9.4 Instruments for Dividing and Anastomosing the Colon and Rectum (Endostaplers)

Stapling devices have been introduced in laparoscopic surgery more than 25 years ago. The Multifire Endo GIA was among the first endostaplers introduced in general surgery [40]. Since then, their application has been evolved to enable quick and safe resection and anastomosis for all colorectal procedures [3, 4]. Endoscopic staplers can be used both for closing and cutting the colon at the resection margins and for creating a lateral-to-lateral anastomosis (Figs. 4.13 and 4.14). They consist of two triple rows of staggered staples, which secure the closing of the intestinal lumen and a blade track, which divides the colon between the staple lines. The knife blade stops one and a half staple length before the end of the staple line to achieve a mucosa-to-mucosa contact.

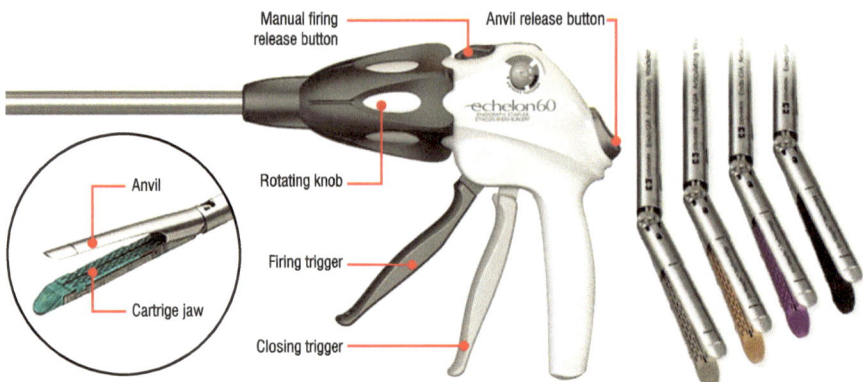

Fig. 4.14 Laparoscopic linear stapler. Echelon Flex TM, Ethicon Endo-Surgery, Inc.

Fig. 4.15 Laparoscopic
anvil grasper

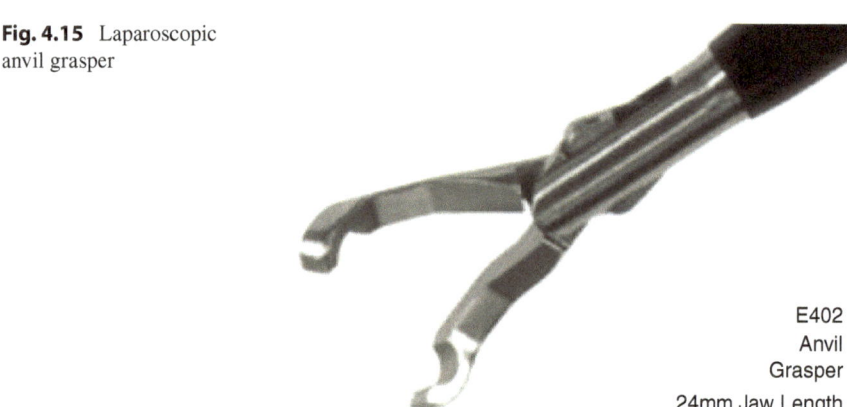

E402
Anvil
Grasper
24mm Jaw Length

The laparoscopic stapling devices are mostly linear. Circular staplers are used in cases of left colonic resections where the anastomosis is performed with the introduction of the stapler from anus. In this case, a conventional circular stapler is used as in open surgery. After division of the distal colon or rectum, the proximal colon is exteriorized through enlargement of one of the trocar sites in the suprapubic region. The colon is then cut and the anvil (Fig. 4.15) is secured in the lumen of the colon with a purse string suture. The colon is then placed in the abdominal cavity. In this case, the anastomosis can be performed under direct vision through the existing incision. Alternatively, the wound is closed and the anastomosis is performed under laparoscopic view. The anvil is grasped with the use of a specially designed laparoscopic anvil grasper or a babcock grasper (Fig. 4.16). After adaption of the anvil to the circular stapler, the stapler is fired [8, 9, 41].

A curved stapler is newly also available in the market (Endo GIA radial reload, Covidien) for cutting of the rectum during an anterior rectum resection (Fig. 4.17). Its configuration is useful in deep anterior resections allowing for weaning appropriate distal margins from the resected tumor. The stapler can be reloaded as the linear staplers.

Fig. 4.16 Babcock
grasper

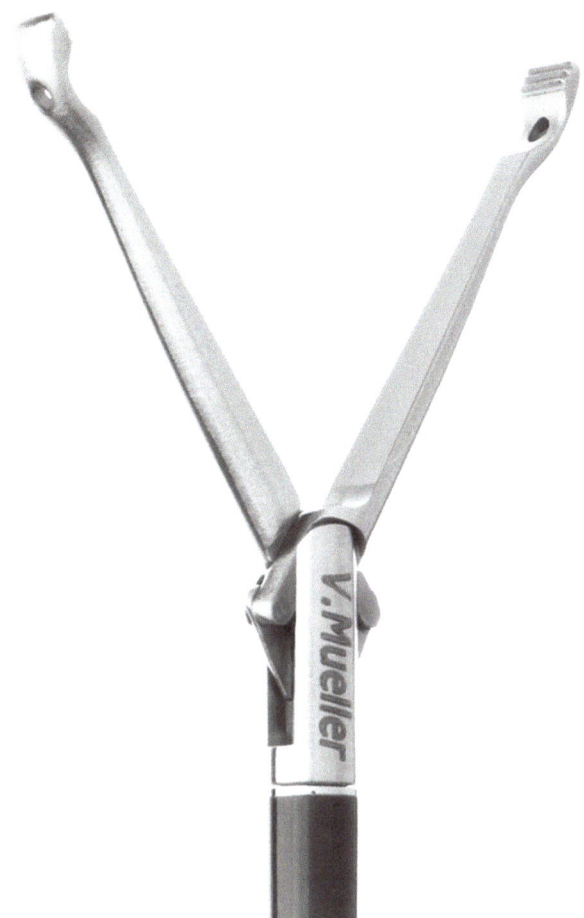

Fig. 4.17 Radial
EndoGIA stapler,
Covidien. (Source: http://
www.medtronic.com/
covidien/products/
surgical-stapling/
endo-gia-radial-reload)

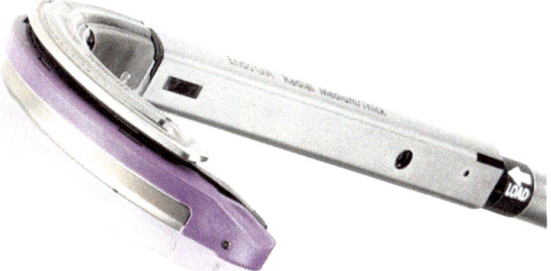

Their length varies between 30 and 60 mm and they are applied through 12 mm laparoscopic cannulas. The length of the cartridge used depends on the length of the planned anastomosis, or the length of the colon to be divided. Laparoscopic stapling devices can be reloaded several times during the same procedure. One has to keep in mind that the length of the colon increases when it becomes compressed between the jaws of the stapler. Furthermore, if multiple firings are required in order to cover the whole length of the colon, the surgeon must include the end of the previous staple line in the new one to avoid leakage. The size of the staples used varies according to the thickness of the intestinal tissue to be closed/divided. Staples are articulated at their handle allowing for 360° rotation. Furthermore, they are also articulated at the base of their body allowing to cut the colon at the desired angle. The surgeon needs to align the stapling device to be able to introduce or remove the staple from the 12 mm cannula. If division and anastomosis of the colon are to be performed extracorporeally, e.g., after a right hemicolectomy, the conventional open stapling devices can be used in the same manner as in open surgery.

4.3.10 Wound Protectors

Wound protectors are used in order to avoid tumor cells deposition at the site of the extraction of the specimen or contamination of the wound in cases of inflammatory disease of the colon (e.g., diverticulitis). Wound protectors consist of one or two flexible rings, which are deformable in order to be introduced in the abdominal cavity through a small incision (Fig. 4.18). This ring is attached to a film, which unfolds covering the whole circumference of the wound. The size of the wound protector used varies according to the size of the incision and the size of the specimen to be

Fig. 4.18 Wound protector. SurgiSleeve. Covidien. (Source: http://www.medtronic.com/covidien/products/trocars-access/surgisleeve-wound-protector)

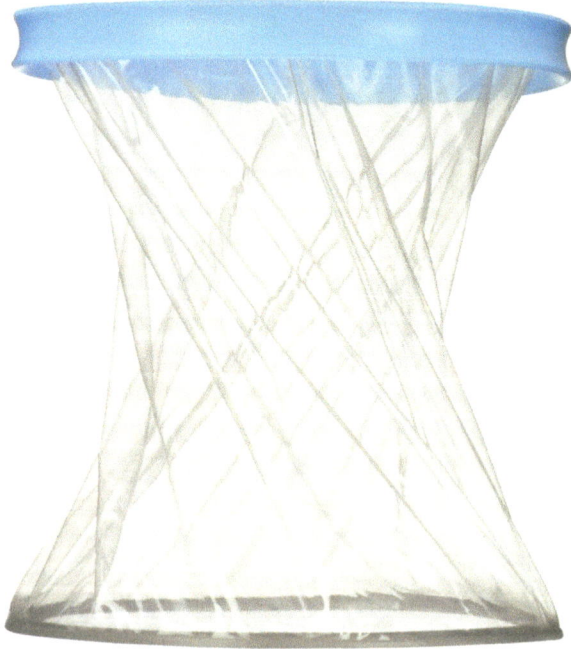

removed [9]. Specimen bags are usually not used in colorectal surgery because the specimens to be removed are long and relatively narrow.

4.4 Conclusions

The availability of the specific instrumentation presented in this chapter is essential for the safe performance of laparoscopic colorectal surgery. The use of a safe mode of energy to achieve adequate and focused hemostasis is the most important component. In addition, the development of specialized instrumentation for the handling, cutting, and anastomosis of the colon can ensure a safe anastomosis. Better visualization of the operative field, through the technological improvements in image processing, is also important for guiding the surgeon through this demanding operation. Further developments are awaited in the ergonomy of the staplers to ensure easier and safer application.

Laparoscopic colorectal surgery has evolved as a result of technological improvements. New instruments, which are continuously improved, contribute to curbing the degree of difficulty of laparoscopic colectomy. Although most surgeons still prefer the open technique, the improvement of surgical instruments gradually but steadily increase the number of surgeons who make laparoscopic colon surgery their first choice of surgical treatment. Increasing, continuous training and skills' improvement is expected to further reinforce the laparoscopic trend in colorectal surgery. Simulation training, education, and best practices, as thoroughly discussed in Chap. 10, in combination with technologically advanced surgical instruments, are the major contributing factors to the improvement of surgical results and the quality of care patients may enjoy.

References

1. Jacobs M, Verdeja JC, Goldstein HS. Minimally invasive colon resection (laparoscopic colectomy). Surg Laparosc Endosc. 1991;1:144–50.
2. Arezzo A, Passera R, Ferri V, Gonella F, Cirocchi R, Morino M. Laparoscopic right colectomy reduces short-term mortality and morbidity. Results of a systematic review and meta-analysis. Int J Color Dis. 2015;30(11):1457–72.
3. Wang CL, Qu G, Xu HW. The short- and long-term outcomes of laparoscopic versus open surgery for colorectal cancer: a meta-analysis. Int J Color Dis. 2014;29(3):309–20.
4. Trastulli S, Cirocchi R, Listorti C, Cavaliere D, Avenia N, Gullà N, Giustozzi G, Sciannameo F, Noya G, Boselli C. Laparoscopic vs open resection for rectal cancer: a meta-analysis of randomized clinical trials. Colorectal Dis. 2012;14(6):e277–96.
5. Blackmore AE, Wong MT, Tang CL. Evolution of laparoscopy in colorectal surgery: an evidence-based review. World J Gastroenterol. 2014;20(17):4926–33.
6. Growing preferences for minimally invasive procedures to drive laparoscopic devices market. 2017. http://www.strategyr.com/MarketResearch/Laparoscopic_Devices_Market_Trends.asp.
7. Young-Fadok TM. Colorectal resections: patient positioning and operating room setup. In: Whelan RL, Fleshman JW, Fowler DL, editors. The SAGES manual of perioperative care in minimally invasive surgery. Heidelberg: Springer Verlag; 2006. p. 150–62.

8. Macaluso A Jr, Larach SW. Laparoscopic Instrumentation. In: MacFayden BJ, editor. Laparoscopic surgery of the abdomen. Heidelberg: Springer Verlag; 2004. p. 335–51.
9. Nakajima K, Milsom JW, Böhm B. Equipment and instrumentation. In: Milsom J, Böhm B, Nakajima K, editors. Laparoscopic colorectal surgery. 2nd ed. Heidelberg: Springer Verlag; 2006. p. 10–29.
10. Gu L, Liu P, Jiang C, Luo M, Xu Q. Virtual digital defogging technology improves laparoscopic imaging quality. Surg Innov. 2015;22(2):171–6. https://doi.org/10.1177/1553350614537564.
11. Ris F, Yeung T, Hompes R, Mortensen NJ. Enhanced reality and intraoperative imaging in colorectal surgery. Clin Colon Rectal Surg. 2015;28(3):158–64.
12. Schols RM, Bouvy ND, van Dam RM, Stassen LP. Advanced intraoperative imaging methods for laparoscopic anatomy navigation: an overview. Surg Endosc. 2013;27(6):1851–9.
13. Park S, Kim NK. The role of robotic surgery for rectal cancer: overcoming technical challenges in laparoscopic surgery by advanced techniques. J Korean Med Sci. 2015;30(7):837–46.
14. Agresta F, Mazzarolo G, Bedin N. Direct trocar insertion for laparoscopy. JSLS. 2012;16(2):255–9. Retrieved from EBSCOhost.
15. Toro A, Mannino M, Cappello G, Di Stefano A, Di Carlo I. Comparison of two entry methods for laparoscopic port entry: technical point of view. Diagn Ther Endosc. 2012;2012:305428, 7 pages. https://doi.org/10.1155/2012/305428.
16. Quilici PJ. New developments in laparoscopy. Burbank, CA: Illustrator - Enid V. Hatton, MA; 1992.
17. Angioli R, Terranova C, Nardone C, Cafà EV, Dmiani P, Portuesi R, Muzii L, Plotti F, Zullo MA, Panici PB. A comparison of three different entry techniques in gynecological laparoscopic surgery: a randomized prospective trial. Eur J Obstet Gynecol Reprod Biol. 2013;171(2):339–42. https://doi.org/10.1016/j.ejogrb.2013.09.012.
18. Alkatout I, Schollmeyer T, Hawaldar NA, Sharma N, Mettler L. Principles and safety measures of Electrosurgery in laparoscopy. JSLS. 2012;16(1):130–9. https://doi.org/10.429 3/108680812X13291597716348.
19. Heijnsdijk EAM, Dankelman J, Gouma DJ. Effectiveness of grasping and duration of clamping using laparoscopic graspers. Surg Endosc. 2002;16(9):1329–31. https://doi.org/10.1007/ s00464-001-9179-2.
20. Geary J. The body electric: an anatomy of the new bionic senses. Rutgers University Press; 2002. p. 130. ISBN 0-8135-3194-2.
21. Suzuki S, Eto K, Hattori A, Yanaga K, Suzuki N. Surgery simulation using patient-specific models for laparoscopic colectomy. Stud Health Technol Informatics. 2007;125(15):464–6. Retrieved from EBSCOhost.
22. Ho Y-H, Tawfik Ashour MA. Techniques for colorectal anastomosis. World J Gastroenterol. 2010;16(13):1610–21. https://doi.org/10.3748/wjg.v16.i13.1610.
23. Szold A. New concepts for a compression anastomosis: superelastic clips and rings. Minim Invasive Ther Allied Technol. 2008;17(3):168–71. https://doi.org/10.1080/13645700802103126.
24. Vilhjalmsson D, Olofsson P, Syk I, Thorlacius H, Grönberg A. The compression anastomotic ring-locking procedure: a novel technique for creating a sutureless colonic anastomosis. Eur Surg Res. 2015;54(3–4):139–47. https://doi.org/10.1159/000368354.
25. Wullstein C, Gross E. Compression anastomosis (AKA-2) in colorectal surgery: results in 442 consecutive patients. Br J Surg. 2000;87(8):1071–5. https://doi. org/10.1046/j.1365-2168.2000.01489x.
26. Debus ES, Sailer M, Geiger D, Dietz UA, Fuchs K-H, Thiede A. Long-term results after 75 anastomoses in the upper extraperitoneal rectum with the biofragmentable anastomosis ring. Dig Surg. 1999;16(1):55–9. https://search-proquest-com.contentproxy.phoenix.edu/docvie w/223608170?accountid=134061
27. Coleman JE. Future developments of the valtrac/biofragmentable anastomosis ring device. In: Engemann R, Thiede A, editors. Compression anastomosis by biofragmentable rings. Berlin: Springer; 1995. p. 156–60. https://doi.org/10.1007/978-3-642-79260-1_27.
28. González-Contreras QH, Jesús-Mosso M, Bahena-Aponte JA, Aldana-Martínez O, Pineda-Solís K, Mejia-Arcadia SN. Colorectal anastomosis using a compression device Anastomosis color-

rectales por compresión utilizando el dispositivo NiTi. Cirugía y Cirujanos. 2016;84(8):482–6. https://doi.org/10.1016/j.circen.2016.11.008.

29. Lee H-Y, Woo J-H, Park S-Y, Kang N-W, Park K-J, Choi H-J. Intestinal anastomosis by use of a memory-shaped compression anastomosis clip (hand CAC 30): early clinical experience. J Kor Soc Coloproctol. 2012;28(2):83–8. https://doi.org/10.3393/jksc.2012.28.2.83.
30. Lee J-Y, Woo JH, Choi HJ, Park KJ, Roh YH, Kim KH, Lee HY. Early experience of the compression anastomosis ring (CARTM 27) in left-sided colon resection. World J Gastroenterol. 2011;17(43):4787–92. https://doi.org/10.3748/wjg.v17.i43.4787.
31. Masoomi H, Luo R, Mills S, Carmichael JC, Senagore AJ, Stamos MJ. Compression anastomosis ring device in colorectal anastomosis: a review of 1,180 patients. Am J Surg. 2013;205(4):447–51. https://doi.org/10.1016/j.amjsurg.2012.03.013.
32. Camran N, Lewis M, King LP Laparoscopic vessel sealing devices. Society of Laparoscopic Surgeons. http://laparoscopy.blogs.com/prevention_management_3/2010/10/laparoscopic-vessel-sealing-devices.html.
33. Böhm B, Milsom JW, Nakajima K. Surgical energy sources. In: Milsom J, Böhm B, Nakajima K, editors. Laparoscopic colorectal surgery. 2nd ed. Heidelberg: Springer Verlag; 2006. p. 30–47.
34. McHoney M. Energy sources in laparoscopic surgery. In: Carachi R, Agarwala S, Bradnock TJ, editors. Basic techniques in pediatric surgery, vol. 2013. Berlin: Springer-Verlag; 2013. p. 539–41.
35. Tou S, Malik AI, Wexner SD, Nelson RL. Energy source instruments for laparoscopic colectomy. Cochrane Database Syst Rev 2011;(5):CD007886.
36. Newcomb WL, Hope WW, Schmelzer TM, et al. Comparison of blood vessel sealing among new electrosurgical and ultrasonic devices. Surg Endosc. 2009;23:90–6.
37. Newman RM, Traverso LW. Principles of laparoscopic hemostasis. In: Scott-Conner CEH, editor. The SAGES manual: fundamentals of laparoscopy, thoracoscopy, and GI endoscopy. 2nd ed. New York: Springer; 2006. p. 49–59.
38. Prabhu AS, Heniford BT. Energy sources in laparoscopy. In: Greene F, Heniford B, editors. Minimally invasive cancer management. New York, NY: Springer; 2009. https://doi.org/10.1007/978-1-4419-1238-1_4.
39. Lorenzo ND, Franceschilli L, Allaix ME, Asimakopoulos A, Sileri P, Gaspari AL. Radiofrequency versus ultrasonic energy in laparoscopic colorectal surgery: a meta-analysis of operative time and blood loss. Surg Endosc. 2012;26(10):2917–24. https://doi.org/10.1007/s00464-012-2285-5.
40. MacFadyen BV, Arregui ME, Eubanks S, Olsen DO, Soper NJ, Wexner SD, Peters JH, Swanström LL, editors. Laparscopic surgery of the abdomen. New York, NY: Springer-Verlag New York; 2004.
41. Slieker JC, Daams F, Mulder IM, Jeekel J, Lange JF. Systematic review of the technique of colorectal anastomosis. JAMA Surg. 2013;148(2):190–201.

Surgical Techniques

5

Sotirios George Panousopoulos
and Constantinos S. Mavrantonis

5.1 Introduction

In this chapter, we will describe the procedures for laparoscopic resection of the colon and rectum, as we perform them routinely in our service. It is important to keep in mind that the described procedures are for malignant disease unless stated otherwise. We have strived to provide a compact, yet complete guide to the full range of colorectal resections and have included considerations on the subject of operative safety. While all these procedures can be performed with significant variation, and indeed have been in the past, this is the extract of our team's experience and our preferred approach.

5.2 Right Hemicolectomy

5.2.1 Pneumoperitoneum, Laparoscopy, and Port Placement

The patient is placed in the supine position. Pneumoperitoneum is established through a 10 mm port placed with an open Hasson technique through the umbilicus. The main monitor is positioned at the patients' right flank area. After laparoscopic

S. G. Panousopoulos
6th Department of Surgery—SRC Center of Excellence for Colorectal Surgery, Hygeia Hospital, Athens, Greece

Director, Simulation Center—NoDE Institute, Athens, Greece

C. S. Mavrantonis (✉)
6th Department of Surgery—SRC Center of Excellence for Colorectal Surgery, Hygeia Hospital, Athens, Greece

Chairman, NoDE Institute, Athens, Greece
e-mail: kmavrantonis@hygeia.gr

© The Editor(s) (if applicable) and The Author(s),
under exclusive license to Springer Nature Switzerland AG 2021
G. Kouraklis, E. (J.) Matsiota (eds.), *Laparoscopic Colon Surgery*,
https://doi.org/10.1007/978-3-030-56728-6_5

83

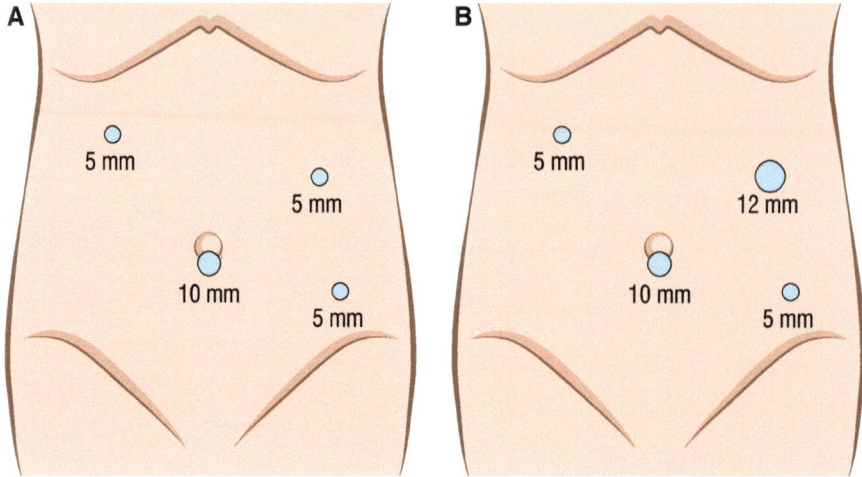

Fig. 5.1 Trocar placement for right colon resection. A = typical, B = for intracorporeal anastomosis. © C.Mavrantonis

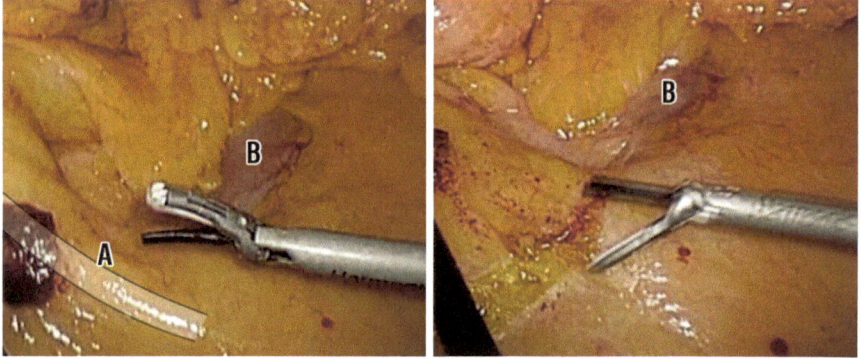

Fig. 5.2 With proper traction, the ileocolic pedicle can be identified as a bowstring in the mesentery (A), immediately inferior to the duodenum (B). © C.Mavrantonis

abdominal exploration, three 5 mm ports are placed as illustrated. Alternatively, if an intracorporeal anastomosis is to be fashioned, a 12 mm port is inserted at the left upper quadrant port site, instead of a 5 mm (Fig. 5.1).

5.2.2 Medial, Ileocolic Vessels

The patient is placed in a steep Trendelenburg position and rotated left. The omentum is placed over the transverse colon and both are retracted cephalad with two 5 mm laparoscopic grasping forceps. Direct handling of the intestinal wall is avoided at all times. The terminal ileum is dropped toward the pelvis, and the small bowel swept to the left. By pulling the ileocecal junction upwards and to the right, the ileocolic vessels are identified inside the mesentery like a bowstring (Fig. 5.2).

A window is opened on the mesentery on either side by use of a direct energy laparoscopic device, and the ileocolic vessels are skeletonized. They are then ligated by use of a laparoscopic clip applier, bipolar diathermy, endoloops, or an endoscopic linear cutter, and divided approximately 1 cm from their origin at the superior mesenteric artery (SMA).

5.2.3   Medial, Middle Colic Vessels

The cut edge of the mesentery is pushed upwards and the underlying duodenum is carefully swept down, meticulously avoiding any thermal injury if diathermy or a direct energy laparoscopic device is utilized (Fig. 5.3).

Laparoscopic shears without diathermy may also be used; however, tedious bleeding may occur. Continuing cephalad, the head of the pancreas is bluntly but gently dissected free in the same manner. This plane of dissection is followed until the middle colic vessels are met. The layers of the transverse mesocolon are dissected and the right branch of the middle colic artery (MCA) is ligated and divided (Fig. 5.4).

Using the direct energy laparoscopic device, the transverse mesocolon is divided starting at the ligation point of the right branch of the MCA, up to the selected site of division of the transverse colon.

5.2.4   Medial, Colon Mobilization

Following the previous dissection plane, the mesocolon is lifted and dissected free from the duodenum and the head of the pancreas. The same dissection plane is gradually extended to the right, under the proximal transverse colon, hepatic flexure, ascending colon, and cecum, meticulously avoiding thermal injuries. As long as the dissection plane remains beneath Toldt's fascia, the right ureter remains out of harm's way.

Fig. 5.3 A = inferior aspect of transverse mesocolon, B = fusion plane between A and underlying peritoneum, C = duodenum, D = head of pancreas.
© C.Mavrantonis

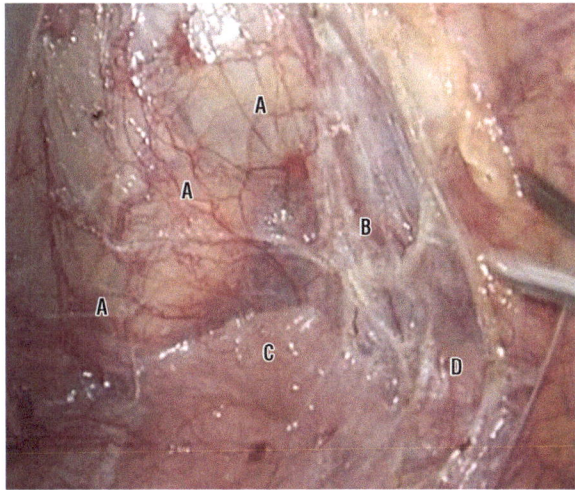

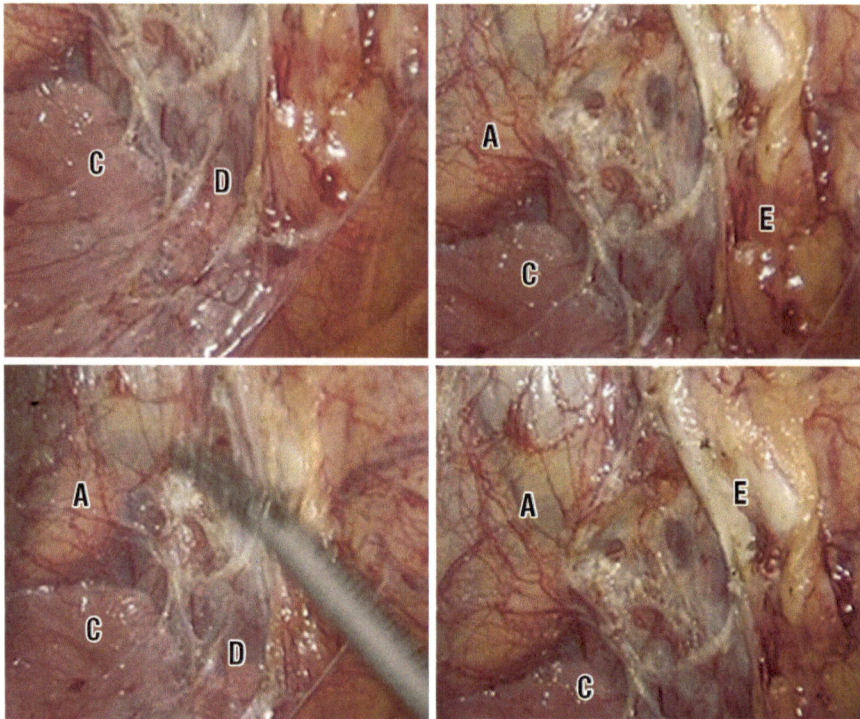

Fig. 5.4 A = inferior aspect of transverse mesocolon, C = duodenum, D = head of pancreas, E = right middle colic vessels. © C.Mavrantonis

5.2.5 Lateral, Ileocecal Mobilization

The terminal ileum is pulled towards the umbilicus with laparoscopic grasping forceps, and its peritoneal attachments are divided with the energy device. A gauze pad placed underneath the ileocecal junction may help identify the already dissected plane and assist completion of mobilization.

5.2.6 Lateral, Right Colon Mobilization

In similar fashion, the ascending colon is freed from its lateral attachments, repositioning the gauze pad as needed, until the proximal portion of the hepatic flexure is freed (Fig. 5.5). To complete mobilization of the hepatic flexure and transverse colon, the patient is repositioned in a reverse Trendelenburg position. The omentum is then dissected free from the stomach, from right to left, up to the point of division of the transverse colon. The omentum is divided with the energy device, to be removed en bloc with the corresponding segment of the colon. Finally, the remaining lateral portion of the hepatic flexure is mobilized (Fig. 5.6).

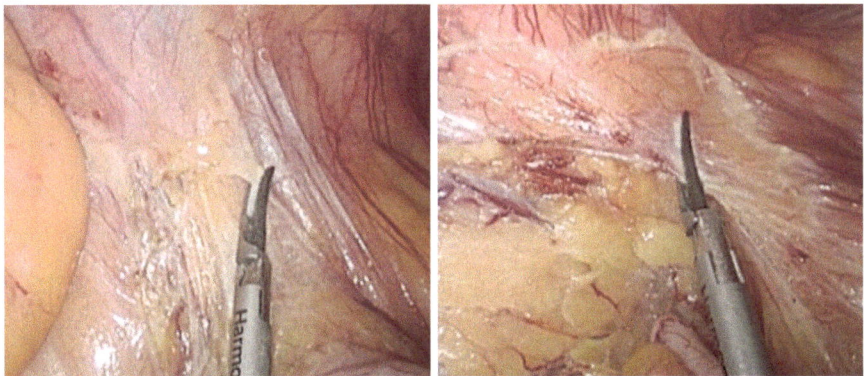

Fig. 5.5 Starting at the ileocecal junction, the lateral attachments of the right colon are divided

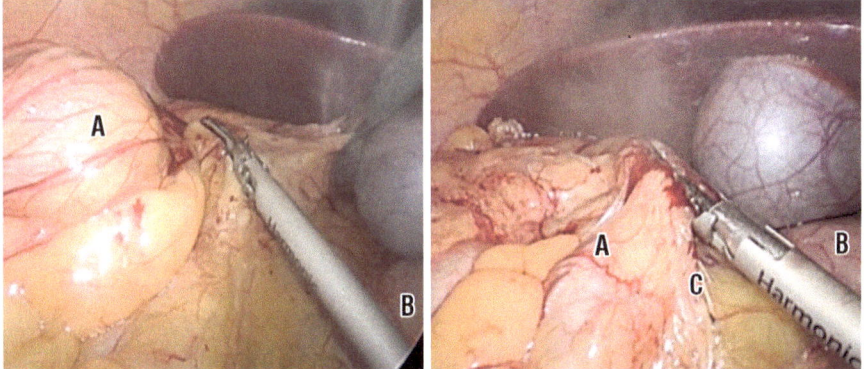

Fig. 5.6 A = colon, B = stomach, C = gastrocolic ligament. © C.Mavrantonis

5.2.7 Resection and Reconstruction

The appendix is secured with a locking grasper, and the patient is returned to a neutral position. A 5–7 cm incision is performed, as an extension of the umbilical port site. The mobilized right colon and terminal ileum are extracted through a wound protector. The terminal ileum is divided 10 cm proximal to the ileocecal junction, with care to ensure adequate blood supply to the stump. Then the transverse colon is divided at least 5 cm distal to the tumor. The ileotransverse anastomosis can be either a hand-sewn or stapled using a linear stapler, as in "open" surgery. Alternatively, the operation may be completed laparoscopically, performing an isoperistaltic anastomosis intracorporeally (Fig. 5.7). The terminal ileum and transverse colon are divided by means of a 60 mm laparoscopic linear cutter. A 1 cm incision is performed on the colic taenia of the transverse colon, 6 cm distal to the stapled stump. Similarly, a 1 cm opening at the staple line of the terminal ileum stump is performed at the antimesenteric edge. The stapler is then introduced through the two puncture sites

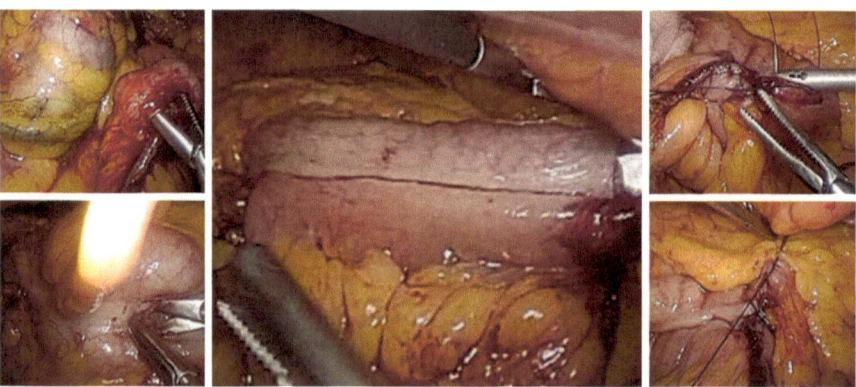

Fig. 5.7 Intracorporeal anastomosis. © C.Mavrantonis

and the jaws are closed. After proper alignment is verified, the stapler is fired. The remaining defect is sutured laparoscopically with a continuous single layer stitch. The specimen is extracted via a small Pfannenstiel incision.

5.3   Extended Right Hemicolectomy

Apart from division of the middle colic vessels, extended right hemicolectomy requires the same strategy and set up as for a right hemicolectomy. In this case, the main trunk of the middle colic vessels is ligated and divided at its origin. The point of distal division for the colon may be the distal transverse colon or the descending colon, if the splenic flexure is to be removed. Mobilization of the splenic flexure is described in "left hemicolectomy."

 Safety Considerations

1. Energy sources generate significant heat. Always keep this in mind and avoid directly handling sensitive tissue such as the intestine or ureters. It is advisable to periodically cool such instruments on fatty tissue or a nearby pool of fluid.

2. Injury to adjacent anatomic features. The SMV, the duodenum and the right ureter are in close proximity to the dissection planes of this operation. To protect the SMV, the GEV and the duodenum, great caution should be exercised during medial dissection. During ligation of the ileocolic pedicle, a small stump should be left, in order to facilitate management of potential bleed.The right ureter may be in danger if the medial plane of dissection of the ileocolic vessels is unclear. In such a case, switch to a lateral approach, identify and trace the ureter before dividing the ileocolic vessels.

5.4   Left Hemicolectomy

5.4.1   Pneumoperitoneum, Laparoscopy, Port Placement

The patient is placed in the modified lithotomy position. Pneumoperitoneum is established through a 10 mm port placed through the umbilicus with the open Hasson technique. The main monitor is positioned at the level of the patient's left knee. After laparoscopic abdominal exploration, one 12 mm port and two 5 mm ports are placed as illustrated (Fig. 5.8).

5.4.2   Medial, Inferior Mesenteric Artery

The patient is placed in a steep Trendelenburg position and rotated right. The omentum is placed over the transverse colon and both are retracted cephalad. The sigmoid colon is retracted out of the pelvis, pulled by the assistant towards the left abdominal wall and cephalad. The sacral promontory is identified and the peritoneum is incised. This incision is continued cephalad over the aorta towards the inferior mesenteric artery (IMA) (Fig. 5.9). Once the IMA is met, dissection is extended towards the lateral aspect of the mesocolon. The avascular plane between the sigmoid mesocolon and Toldt's fascia is entered and the left ureter is visualized (Fig. 5.10). The IMA is then skeletonized, ligated, and divided, approximately 1 cm from its origin, by use of bipolar diathermy, clips, or vascular endoscopic linear stapler. During division of the IMA, the ureter must remain under direct vision at all

Fig. 5.8   Trocar placement for left colon resection. © C.Mavrantonis

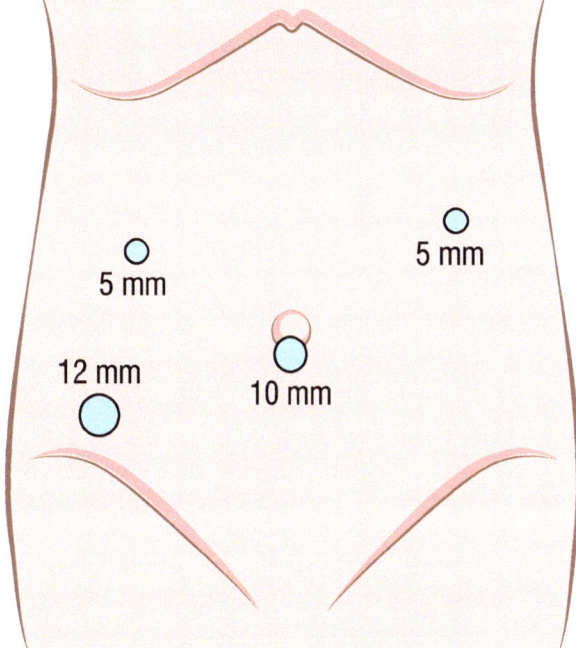

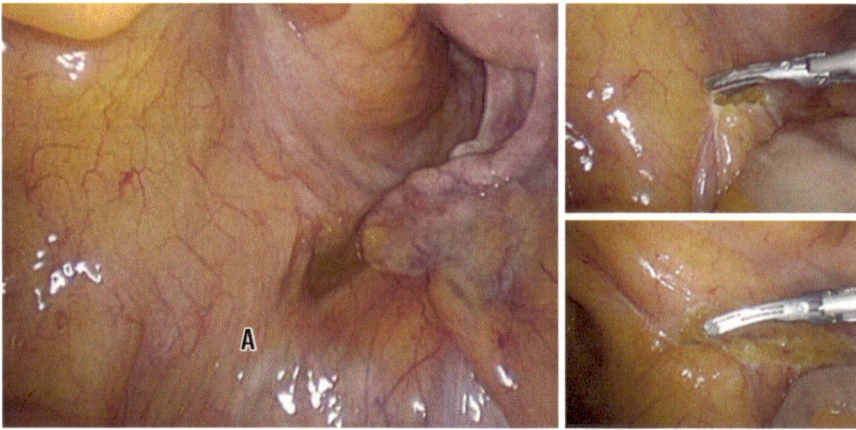

Fig. 5.9 A = sacral promontory. © C.Mavrantonis

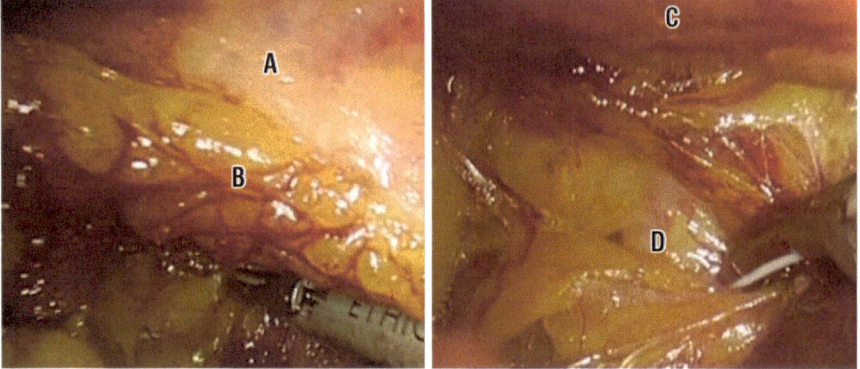

Fig. 5.10 A = right aspect of sigmoid mesocolon, B = dissected surface of the sigmoid mesocolon, C = left (inferior) aspect of sigmoid mesocolon, D = left ureter. © C.Mavrantonis

times. The medial aspect of the mesocolon is further incised from the ligated IMA to the chosen site of proximal division of the colon. The inferior mesenteric vein is met, ligated, and divided.

5.4.3   Splenic Flexure Mobilization

The sigmoid and descending colon are freed of their lateral attachments, starting at the point where division of Toldt's white line meets the previously dissected medial plane. This can be facilitated by positioning a gauze pad through the medial plane adjacent to the visualized left ureter. Dissection is then carried cephalad to the splenic flexure. Approaching the spleen, care should be taken not to exert excessive traction on the descending colon, in order to avoid avulsion injury. When this is completed,

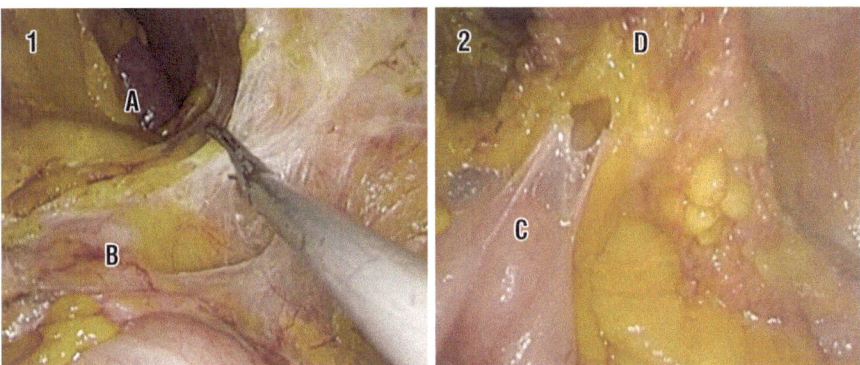

Fig. 5.11 1, Lateral mobilization of descending colon (A = spleen, B = descending colon) 2, Entry into the lesser sac (C = transverse colon, D = omentum). © C.Mavrantonis

the patient is brought to a reverse Trendelenburg position. The assistant's laparo-scopic grasper is removed and the surgeon extends his/her right hand across the patient to insert the energy device through the freed port. Using this, the lesser sac is entered at the middle to distal one-third of the transverse colon, and the omentum is dissected free of the colon's superior border (Fig. 5.11). This dissection continues until the splenic flexure is free of the omentum and spleen. It is then retracted towards the pelvis while the remaining attachments to the retroperitoneum are divided.

5.4.4   Distal Division of the Colon

Following complete mobilization of the splenic flexure, descending colon, and sig-moid colon, the patient is returned to the Trendelenburg position and the surgeon moves back to the two right-side ports. The rectosigmoid junction is now prepared for dissection. Starting at the level of the sacral promontory, the presacral space is entered and dissected up to the peritoneal reflection, which is opened circumferen-tially. Using a direct energy laparoscopic device, the upper mesorectum is gradually divided until the posterior wall of the bowel is freed from any mesorectal tissue. Once the bowel wall is completely free of any mesorectal fat, it is divided using an endoscopic linear stapling device (Fig. 5.12).

5.4.5   Resection and Reconstruction

The patient is returned to a neutral position, and a 5–7 cm Pfannenstiel incision is made. The mobilized colon is extracted through a wound protector. The colonic lumen is divided, generally including the mobilized splenic flexure within the speci-men. Having verified that the stump is well vascularized, the anvil of a 29 mm circular stapler is secured at the cut edge with a purse string suture, and the colon is returned to the abdomen. The Pfannenstiel incision is closed and pneumoperitoneum

Fig. 5.12 A = peritoneal reflection, B = upper mesorectum. © C. Mavrantonis

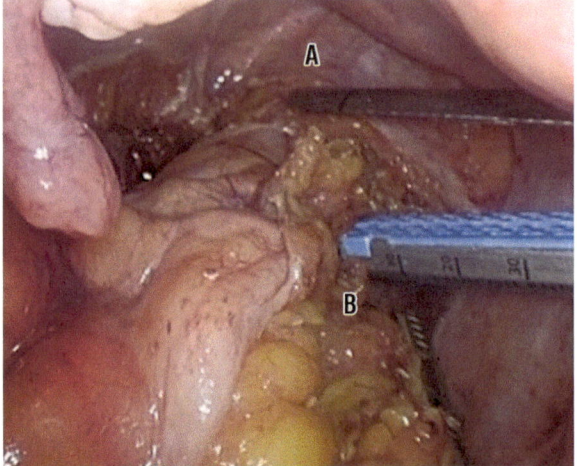

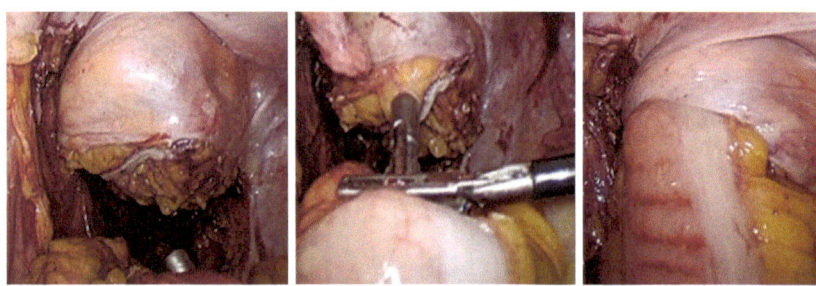

Fig. 5.13 Circular stapler anastomosis and air- test. © C.Mavrantonis

reestablished. The patient is once more placed in the steep Trendelenburg position and rotated right. The circular stapler is introduced transanally, to gently press against the rectal stump suture line. The circular stapler's trocar is advanced through the staple line and the anvil is laparoscopically coupled to the stapler (Fig. 5.13). Orientation of the proximal stump is checked for potential rotation, the stapler is tightened, and, after confirming that the anastomosis will be tension-free, the stapler is fired and removed. The pelvis is filled with saline and the anastomosis is tested by insufflating air through the anus. The "doughnuts" are retrieved from the stapler, checked for integrity, and sent along with the specimen for pathology review.

5.5   Sigmoid Colectomy for Diverticular Disease

Sigmoid colectomy for diverticular disease follows the same steps as in left hemicolectomy. However, as this is a benign disease, high ligation of the IMA is unnecessary and discouraged, in order to keep the hypogastric nerve plexus out of harm's way. Moreover, splenic flexure mobilization may, occasionally, prove unnecessary.

Safety Considerations

1. Energy sources generate significant heat. Always keep this in mind and avoid directly handling sensitive tissue such as the intestine or ureters. It is advisable to periodically cool such instruments on fatty tissue or a nearby pool off luid.

2. Injury to adjacent anatomic features. The Hypogastric Nerve Plexus (HNP), the left ureter and the spleen are in close proximity to the dissection planes of this operation. To protect the HNP, dissect the IMA atleast 1cm from its origin. The ureter is best preserved if identified before IMA division, especially if a stapling device is to be used for ligation.The spleen should be handled gently, and traction to the colon and/or omentum should be cautious.

2. Spatial awareness during reconstruction. During anastomosis, the proximal stump may rotate along its axis. After initial correction, itis advisable to reevaluate before firing the circular stapler.

5.6   Low Anterior Resection, Total Mesorectal Excision

The procedure described here is the laparoscopic component of three different operations: low anterior resection, intersphincteric resection, and abdominoperineal resection. Depending on the operation, resection and reconstruction vary. Figure 5.14 illustrates the three different resection paths.

5.6.1   Pneumoperitoneum, Laparoscopy, Port Placement

As per left hemicolectomy. If, however, an intersphincteric resection is planned, all three working ports may be of a 5 mm diameter (see "Left Hemicolectomy" above).

5.6.2   Medial, Inferior Mesenteric Artery

As per left hemicolectomy—see "Left Hemicolectomy" above.

5.6.3   Splenic Flexure Mobilization

As per left hemicolectomy—see "Left Hemicolectomy" above.

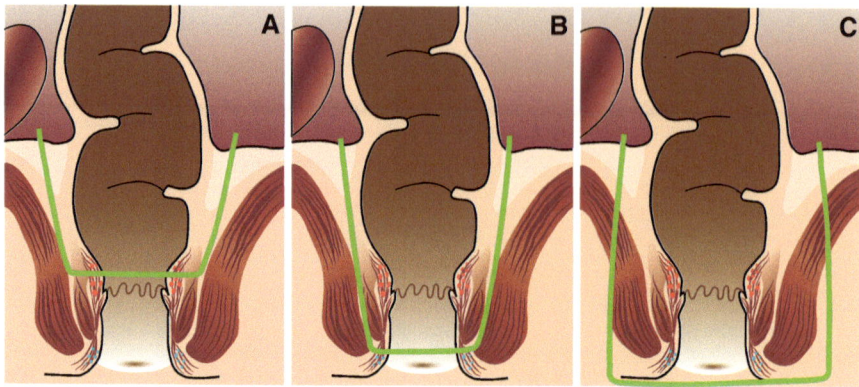

Fig. 5.14 A = low anterior resection, B = intersphincteric resection, C = abdominoperineal resection (Armin Kübelbeck, with permission CC-BY-SA)

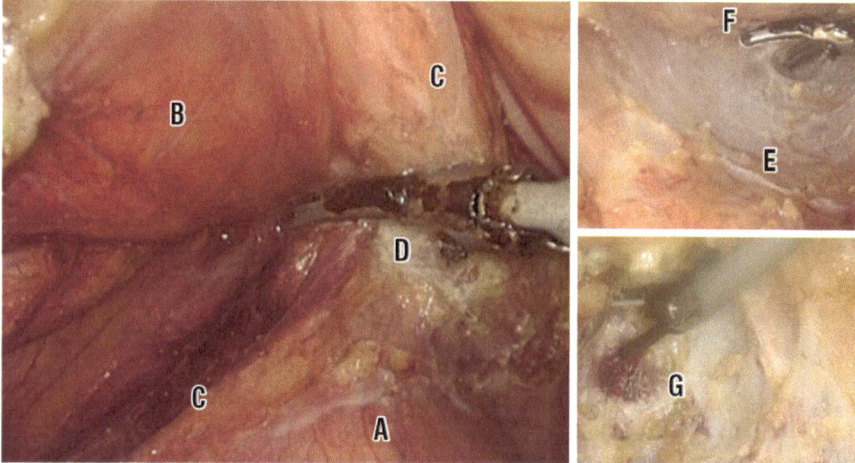

Fig. 5.15 A = sacral promontory, B = sigmoid mesocolon (posterior aspect), C = incised sigmoid mesocolon (medial aspect), D = entry into the presacral space, E = sacral fascia, F = mesorectum (posterior aspect), G = pelvic floor. © C.Mavrantonis

5.6.4   Total Mesorectal Excision

Starting at the sacral promontory, the presacral space is entered. Posterior dissection of the mesorectum can be accomplished along the avascular plane between the sacral fascia and the posterior mesorectal fascia (Fig. 5.15). Dissection along this avascular plane is performed with laparoscopic shears, a direct energy laparoscopic device, or a laparoscopic hook electrode. Accidental entry into the sacral fascia may

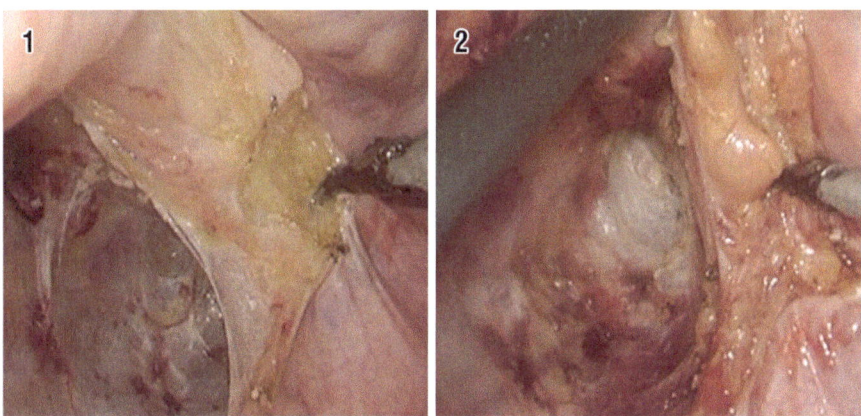

Fig. 5.16 Division of the lateral stalks (shown right side). © C.Mavrantonis

Fig. 5.17 A = prostate,
B = rectal wall.
© C.Mavrantonis

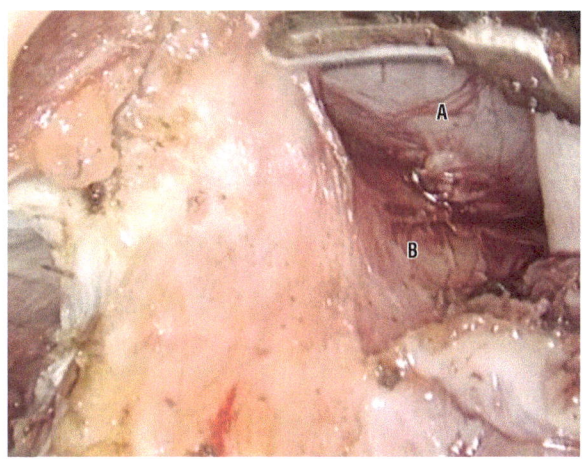

lead to significant venous bleeding, while entry into the mesorectum anteriorly will result in a poor-quality resection from an oncologic standpoint. Next, the lateral stalks are divided close to the rectum, and dissection extends to the anterior rectal wall (Fig. 5.16). After dividing the anterior peritoneal reflection, the anterior wall of the rectum is slowly dissected free from the posterior aspect of the vagina in female patients, or the seminal vesicles and prostate in male patients (Fig. 5.17). Succession from posterior to lateral to anterior dissection is repeated as needed in order to reach the pelvic floor and completely mobilize the mesorectum, down to and including its tail (Fig. 5.18). This way, the rectum may be divided with an endoscopic linear stapler at the level of the anorectal junction (Fig. 5.18), or transanally with subsequent specimen retrieval through the anus.

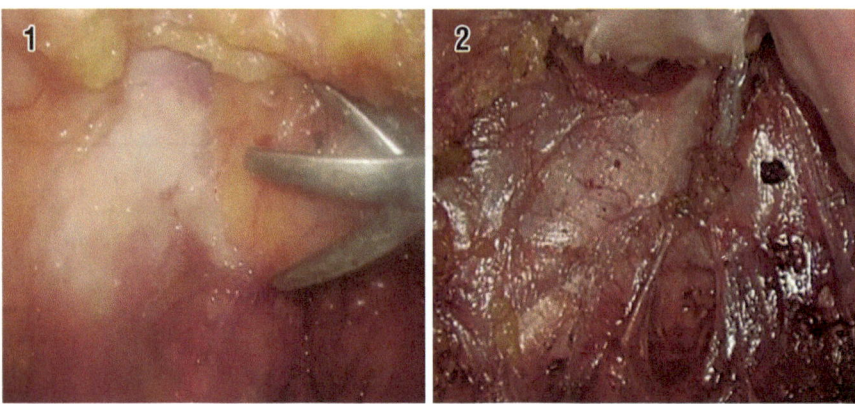

Fig. 5.18 1 = dissection of the mesorectal tail using laparoscopic shears, 2 = the rectum divided at the levator ani level. © C.Mavrantonis

5.6.5 Resection and Reconstruction

For a low anterior resection, after division of the lumen at the anorectal junction with an endoscopic linear stapler, the patient is returned to a neutral position, and a 5–7 cm Pfannenstiel incision is made. The mobilized colon is extracted through a wound protector. The point of proximal division is identified, the lumen is divided, and the specimen is removed. The anvil of a 29 mm circular stapler is secured to the well-vascularized stump with a purse string suture and returned into the abdomen. The Pfannenstiel incision is closed and pneumoperitoneum reestablished. The patient is once more placed in a steep Trendelenburg position and rotated right. The circular stapler is introduced transanally and its trocar is advanced through the staple line. The anvil is laparoscopically advanced down the pelvis with an anvil grasper and coupled to the stapler. Having established correct orientation and absence of tension, the stapler is tightened, fired, and removed. The remainder of the procedure is as per left hemicolectomy (see "Left Hemicolectomy" above). A loop ileostomy is matured at the preoperatively marked site, at the right lateral abdominal wall. A suction drain is placed in the pelvis.

For an ultra-low or an intersphincteric resection, the abdominal field is covered, and the surgeon moves to the perineum. The intersphincteric plane is entered, beginning at the intersphincteric groove or above the dentate line, depending on the tumor site. A combination of monopolar and bipolar diathermy facilitates hemostasis. Dissection continues circumferentially until the pelvic floor is breached at the levator ani muscles and the two dissection planes meet. The mobilized rectum and inner sphincter are brought through the external sphincter lumen. The colon is divided extracorporeally, and a hand-sewn coloanal anastomosis is fashioned, ideally after construction of a colonic J-pouch. A covering loop ileostomy is fashioned at the right lateral abdominal wall. A suction drain is placed in the pelvis.

For an abdominoperineal resection (APR), the laparoscopic phase of the operation concludes with division of the descending colon at the appropriate site, by use of a laparoscopic linear stapler. The abdominal field is covered and the surgeon moves to the perineum. The operation is completed as per the open APR technique and the perineal wound is closed. Pneumoperitoneum is reestablished and the colonic stump is externalized to create an end left lateral abdominal wall colostomy, at the preoperatively marked site.

5.7 Total Proctocolectomy with Ileoanal J-Pouch Anastomosis

5.7.1 Pneumoperitoneum, Laparoscopy, Port Placement

The patient is placed in the modified lithotomy position. Pneumoperitoneum is established through the umbilicus, where a 10 mm port is placed. The main monitor is positioned at the patient's right flank and the surgeon stands at the patient's left. After laparoscopic abdominal exploration, one 12 mm port and three 5 mm ports are placed as illustrated (Fig. 5.19).

5.7.2 Right Colon

The operation begins as per right hemicolectomy (see "Right Hemicolectomy" above). The medial to lateral approach is employed. After dissection of the ileocolic

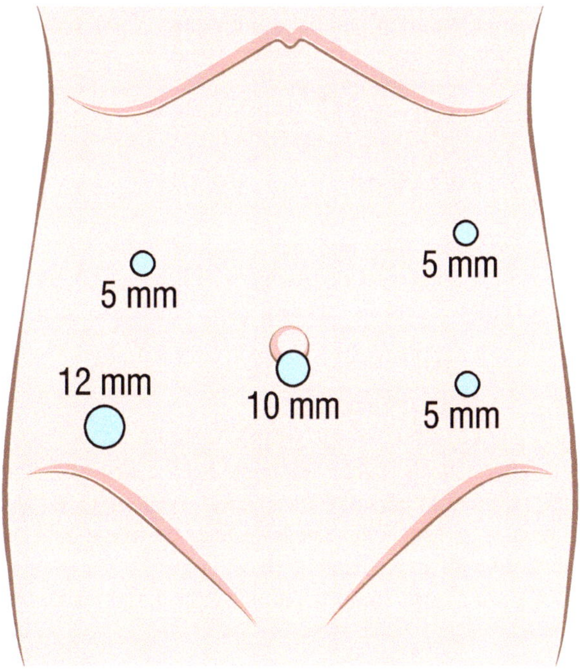

Fig. 5.19 Trocar placement for total proctocolectomy. © C.Mavrantonis

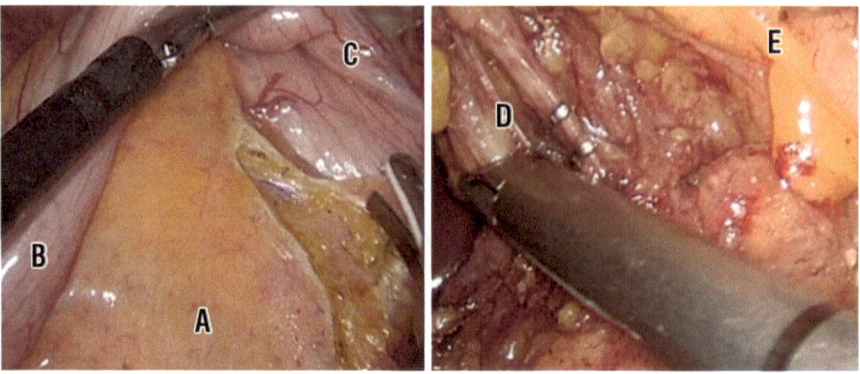

Fig. 5.20 Vascular division close to the colon. A = ileocolic pedicle, B = terminal ileum, C = cecum, D = middle colic vessels, E = transverse colon. Trocar Placement for Total Proctocolectomy. © C.Mavrantonis

pedicle, the ileocolic vessels are not ligated at their origin. Dissection continues to the bowel wall and only tributaries irrigating the colon are ligated (Fig. 5.20), in order to preserve vascularization of the full length of the terminal ileum.

Similarly, the middle colic vessels may be divided close to the colon, thus avoiding the risk involved in a complete mesocolic excision (Fig. 5.20). In order to preserve the omentum, it is dissected free of the transverse colon. When this dissection has reached the mid-transverse colon, the main monitor is repositioned at the patients left flank and the surgeon moves to the patient's right. Dissection continues along the length of the distal transverse colon, leading to splenic flexure mobilization, from right to left. Having freed the splenic flexure, mobilization proceeds along the descending colon.

5.7.3   Left Colon

The procedure now continues as per left hemicolectomy (see "Left Hemicolectomy" above). After dissection, the IMA is ligated and divided at its bifurcation. The sigmoid colon is mobilized in the above-described manner.

5.7.4   Rectal Excision

At this point, the entire colon has been mobilized. The next step is mobilization of the rectum, as per total mesorectal excision (see "Low Anterior Resection, Total Mesorectal Excision" above). Once the rectum is fully mobilized, the lumen is divided with an endoscopic linear stapler at the level of the anorectal junction, if an ileo pouch–anal anastomosis (IPAA) is to be fashioned.

5.7.5 Resection and Reconstruction

The patient is returned to a neutral position and the mobilized colon is extracted through the ileostomy site. The ileum is divided right at the ileocecal junction. Once the length of the ileum is considered adequate to fashion a tension-free pouch anal anastomosis, a 15–20 cm in length ileal J-pouch is formed with consecutive deployment of a 10 cm linear stapler. A purse string suture at the linear stapler opening, secures in place the anvil of a 29 mm circular stapler. The ileum is returned to the abdomen. Pneumoperitoneum is reestablished and the patient is once more placed in a steep Trendelenburg position and rotated right. The circular stapler is gently introduced transanally and the trocar is advanced through the stump's suture line. The anvil is laparoscopically advanced down the pelvis with an anvil grasper and coupled with the stapler. In order to avoid twisting of the mesentery, orientation and alignment of the J-pouch are thoroughly checked and confirmed, before carrying out the anastomosis. When this evaluation is complete, the stapler is fired. The anastomosis is tested by air insufflation, as per low anterior resection. A loop ileostomy is matured through the opening used for the specimen extraction. A suction drain is placed in the pelvis.

Complications in Laparoscopic Colorectal Surgery

6

Chrysanthi Aggeli, Alexander-Michael Nixon, and Georgios N. Zografos

6.1 Introduction

Colorectal surgery is considered one of the central pillars of general surgery and its scope has expanded to treat many common disorders such as colon cancer, ulcerative colitis, inflammatory bowel disease, mechanical bowel obstruction, recurrent diverticulitis, injury, and ischemia. In certain cases, the procedures employed can be technically challenging and frequently require considerable reconstruction of the gastrointestinal tract.

Since its advent in the 1990s, the use of minimally invasive surgical techniques has increased in colorectal surgery. Multiple studies have demonstrated improved short-term and long-term outcomes when compared to open surgery [1, 2]. Laparoscopic colorectal procedures have a steep learning curve, especially when considering the parameters of operative time and conversion as indicators of improvement. A surgeon needs to perform approximately 30–70 cases to achieve technical proficiency [3]. If readmission rates and major complications are also considered as indicators then the learning curve becomes even steeper [4]. Despite difficulties in establishing reproducible learning curves, every specialized center has employed minimally invasive techniques as a safe method of care over the past 10–15 years.

Laparoscopic colorectal surgery is qualitatively associated with the same type of operative risks and complications as open surgery. Resection and reconstruction of the gastrointestinal tract at any level may be associated with postoperative hemorrhage, anastomotic leaks, and abdominal wall hernias. In experienced hands, however, the incidence of other common complications of open surgery such as bowel obstruction is reported to be less frequent in laparoscopic colectomy [5].

C. Aggeli · A.-M. Nixon · G. N. Zografos (✉)
Third Department of Surgery, General Hospital of Athens "G. Gennimatas", Athens, Greece

Although some complications associated with colorectal surgery have been reduced with the use of laparoscopy, including respiratory sequela, venous thromboembolism, and surgical site infection, other problems such as anastomotic leakage and bleeding persist, albeit with less frequency regardless of the approach used, and there seems to be no discernible difference in mortality compared to laparotomy when patients are properly stratified for risk factors [6].

Complications can be divided to those that are unique to laparoscopic surgery and are the result of the equipment employed and conventional complications that are common to open colorectal surgery. The risk of certain major complications such as major vessel injury or bowel injury is similar to either laparoscopic or open colectomy technique.

Although laparoscopic colectomy is associated with a reduction in certain postoperative complications such as respiratory compromise and postprocedural pain compared to traditional approaches, there seems to be a loss of these benefits if the time of the procedure is too long [7]. "Heroic" attempts in performing the whole surgical procedure laparoscopically can have a direct adverse effect on the outcome. The surgeon must be willing to proceed with a conversion procedure, if there is no discernible progress during laparoscopy. It is our opinion that this mentality and attitude safeguards the surgeon and the patient against several pitfalls.

6.2   Surgical Complications

Complications can be broadly divided into surgical and medical complications. Surgical complications are those that can be directly associated with the surgical technique employed during the procedure. These can be identified as intraoperative (e.g., major vascular injury) or can evolve at the postoperative phase (e.g., thermal injury to the duodenum or anastomotic leak). Medical complications are not directly attributed to the surgical maneuvers during the procedure but can be the result of other factors such as anesthesia management and coagulation mechanism dysfunction (e.g., respiratory complications or deep venous thrombosis). In this chapter, we focus mainly on the differences between surgical complications when comparing laparoscopic colorectal surgery to open surgery.

6.3   Complications Related to the Laparoscopic Technique

There are two major differences between laparoscopic procedures and open abdominal surgery. The first difference relates to the abdominal access and the second is the establishment of pneumoperitoneum. These complications were primarily observed during the early years of laparoscopic surgery and certain early conclusions may not be applicable today. Experience and refinement of equipment have made most of the complications related to these issues exceedingly improbable but not impossible and we will review them both in this chapter.

6.3.1   Complications Related to Initial Abdominal Entry

There are three basic modes to enter the abdominal cavity to establish pneumoperitoneum in laparoscopic surgery:

(a) Blind insertion of a primary port without creation of pneumoperitoneum.
(b) Creation of the pneumoperitoneum with a Veress needle (closed technique).
(c) Small incision and direct visualization while placing the primary port (Hasson technique).

All these techniques are associated with varying degrees of complications. Despite anecdotal evidence and small-scale studies, no significant differences in major complications (visceral or vascular injuries) seem to exist when comparing open to closed techniques, but closed techniques have been associated with a higher likelihood of failure of entry [8]. The lack of noticeable differences in major complications could be a reflection of the limitations in the design of these studies. At our institution, we usually prefer the open technique, which allows direct visualization of the port insertion site. This is of special importance for patients with a prior history of abdominal procedures where intra-abdominal adhesions may render port insertion risky. Even though there does not seem to be compelling evidence in the literature review due to the rarity of major complications, the authors believe that visceral injury is more readily identifiable with the open technique and thus amenable to immediate management. However, in our experience, there are occasional cases where closed techniques may be preferred, over the Hasson technique. One such case is when dealing with a morbidly obese patient. The excessive subcutaneous tissue can render the open technique challenging and time-consuming.

Veress needle insertion and that of the first port are potentially dangerous steps in laparoscopic surgery as access is accomplished blindly. Historically, this first step had been considered a common cause of major vascular injury [9]. This however has not been substantially proven in subsequent reports. Insertion of the Veress needle should be performed perpendicularly to the abdominal wall and in a controlled fashion. Steady force should be applied and the surgeon should be prepared to immediately retract the needle if sudden loss of tissue resistance is felt. In this fashion, major vascular injury can be avoided. In cases of previous laparotomy, the surgeon should assume the presence of intra-abdominal adhesions and possible distortion of the normal anatomy. In these patients, the use of the Veress needle should be avoided.

Insertion of the other ports is done under direct vision in an attempt to avoid injuries. Even though surgical textbooks provide standard points of insertion for specific procedures based on anatomical landmarks, one usually places the working ports by transillumination[1] and palpation of the abdominal wall based on each patient's body habitus. In an attempt to avoid undue resistance from the ports, they

---

[1] Transillumination is a test where bright light is used to see the structure of an organ or cavity.

should be placed in the direction of the operating field. When possible they should be spaced apart at least 5 cm in order to avoid interference and to enjoy full range of motion. If deemed necessary, additional ports can be placed during the procedure in a similar fashion.

During placement of the other ports, the port type could be another predisposing factor in minor and major complications. There seems to be limited evidence that cutting compared to radially expanding ports are associated with higher incidence of port site bleeding [10]. These observations are rarely documented during laparoscopic procedures and therefore there are no good quality data to support this claim. Port site bleeding is referred to as a minor complication, which is obviously true when compared to visceral or major vascular injuries. It should be noted, though, that this complication can occasionally be difficult to manage, leading to increased operating time and frustration.

A rarely mentioned issue in laparoscopic surgery is the size of the skin incisions. When performing a laparoscopic operation, the skin incisions should follow a "Goldilocks principle" meaning that they should be neither too large nor too small. Very small incisions render the insertion of the port much too difficult, as it creates the need of an increased outside pressure for the introduction of the port. Increased tension will result in poor cosmesis and, in extreme cases, skin necrosis. On the other hand, too large incisions result in gas loss, port dislocation, and more trauma.

6.3.2   Complications Related to Pneumoperitoneum

Incorrect insufflation of CO_2 into tissue compartments other than the abdominal cavity such as the adipose tissue or preperitoneal space can lead to significant intra or postoperative hypercapnia and clinically significant subcutaneous emphysema. Complications such as these may occur because of improper use of the laparoscope as a lever, an excessive number of ports, and improper placement technique [11]. Misplacement of the Veress needle has also been cited as a frequent cause. The introduction of electronic insufflators equipped with automatic flow stop and anesthesiological monitoring devices have diminished clinical consequences of the complication. Pneumoperitoneum has been observed to cause changes in other physiological parameters such as intracranial and intrathoracic pressures [12]. The clinical significance of these alterations is not well understood but it seems that prolonged pneumoperitoneum could pose dangers for high-risk patients (e.g., recent history of head trauma) [13].

6.4   Vascular Injuries

Blood vessels' injury most commonly occurs during abdominal access but it can also happen during the dissection phase. It can be grouped into minor and major vessel injuries.

6.4.1 Minor Vessel Injury

Vascular complications most commonly result from laceration of minor vessels. Although the injured vessel is considered minor, these injuries are sometimes the cause of conversion to an open procedure or reoperation. The bleeding site can be coagulated or clipped. During initial abdominal entry, the omental and mesenteric vessels are most commonly injured but the most common vascular injury is laceration of the inferior epigastric artery during the placement of lateral ports in the lower abdomen [14]. Cutting ports with sharp blades are probably more likely to injure vessels compared with smooth, conical ones that push the vessel out of the way; however, there is a lack of good quality data to substantiate this claim [10]. A basic principle of trauma surgery is that hemostasis is harder to achieve in partial lacerations of minor and medium size arteries compared to complete lacerations. Even though it may seem counterintuitive, partial lacerations of the inferior epigastric artery vessels may be more challenging to control because spasm of the vessel can exacerbate the laceration leading to greater blood loss. In our experience, injury of the epigastric vessels is a very rare event, which can be usually prevented by avoiding placement of the port along the vessels' anticipated course between the rectus abdominis muscle and the posterior lamella of the sheath. Similar to the inferior epigastric vessels, other abdominal wall vessels can be injured, particularly if the port is not placed under direct vision, and if secondary ports are placed without prior transillumination of the abdominal wall to identify their presence. Bleeding from a port site may only become evident after completion of the procedure and removal of the port due to a tamponade effect.

Therefore, port site inspection is necessary during placement and after the completion of the procedure during removal. In most cases, electrocoagulation suffices but more extensive bleeding may require other measures. A Foley catheter can be inserted to offer a temporary tamponade effect. In challenging cases, a suture can be placed through the port site using an endo-close device. In our experience, this measure is adequate in these scenaria.

Delayed bleeding can occur after the patient has been transferred from the operating room, typically within 1 h. Patients can present hemodynamic instability due to significant blood loss from a port site that bleeds internally. However, delayed abdominal wall hematomas can appear 2 or 3 days after surgery. Clinical manifestations include abdominal wall pain, abdominal wall or flank ecchymosis, and external bleeding from a port site. Patients with an abdominal wall hematoma from laparoscopic access, who are hemodynamically stable and with no signs of hematoma expansion, can be managed conservatively. The hematoma may drain spontaneously through one or more port sites. Intervention is indicated if the hematoma expands, the patient becomes hemodynamically unstable, or the hematoma becomes infected. For some patients, percutaneous embolization of the bleeding vessel may be an option; however, rapidly expanding hematomas leading to hemodynamic instability or infected hematomas are more effectively managed using an open surgical approach.

6.4.2 Major Vessel Injury

Major vessel injury is a rare but potentially life-threatening complication. Advances in technology and experience with laparoscopic surgery have significantly reduced the incidence of these complications. Traditionally, the aorta and the inferior vena cava are considered to be the major vessels most commonly injured during laparoscopic procedures in general [15]. A major vascular injury may occur due to the proximity of important vascular structures to the anterior abdominal wall. In the case of thin individuals, the distance from the anterior abdominal wall to the aorta can be as little as 2 cm (Fig. 6.1).

In laparoscopic colorectal surgery, the iliac vessels are in close proximity to the operating field and thus vulnerable to inadvertent injury [16]. The distal aorta, which lies directly beneath the umbilicus, and right common iliac artery, which crosses the midline, are each particularly prone to injury (Fig. 6.2). Injury of the aorta or iliac vessels during abdominal access can lead to severe hemorrhage and death unless prompt vascular control and repair are managed. Major vascular injuries are almost always recognized immediately because of pooling of blood in the abdominal cavity. In certain cases, bleeding may become evident later because of sequestration of blood in other compartments such as the mesentery or retroperitoneum. When major vessel compromise is observed, immediate action is required. Laparotomy is performed with a midline incision, and direct pressure is applied to the offended vessel. In the event that a vessel injury cannot be identified then packing with laparotomy pads is an acceptable temporary measure. If an injury to a major vessel is found, the surgeon must decide whether to proceed with ligation, primary repair, or interposition graft placement. In rare cases, laparoscopic repair has been performed but the authors do not recommend this as a first-line approach.

Fig. 6.1 Folley catheter

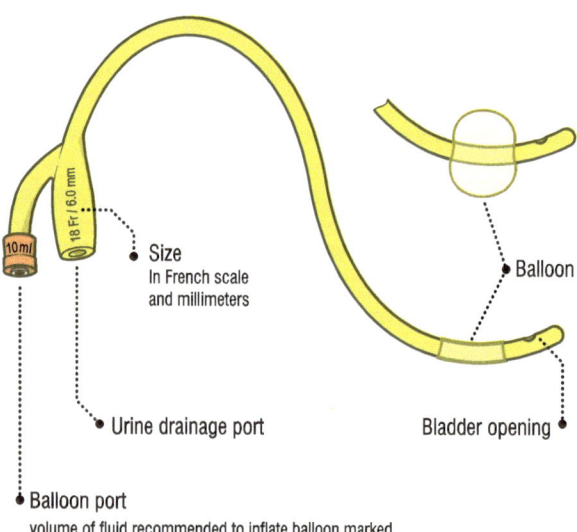

Size
In French scale
and millimeters

Balloon

Urine drainage port

Bladder opening

Balloon port
volume of fluid recommended to inflate balloon marked

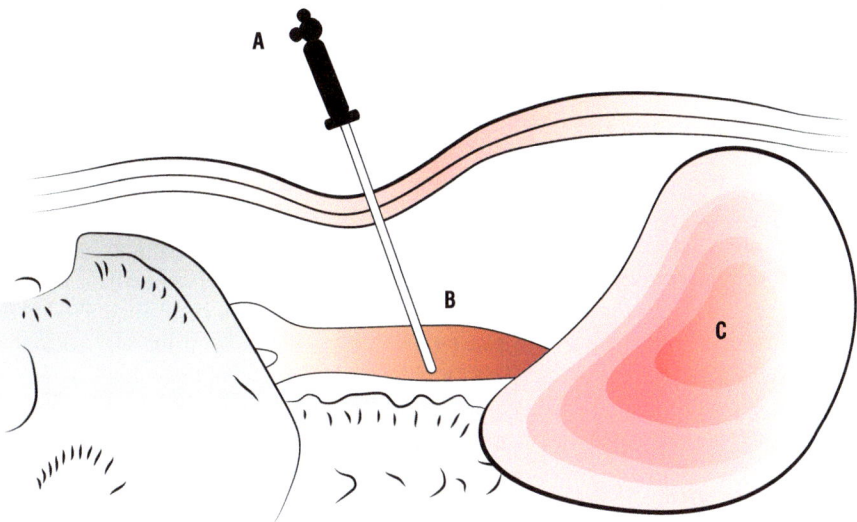

Fig. 6.2 Anterior abdominal wall and aorta distance

Application of pressure over a large area is virtually impossible laparoscopically and major bleeding usually obscures the laparoscopic operating field increasing the likelihood of inadvertent injury during tissue manipulation.

Damage to major veins can be especially problematic due to their thin wall and in certain cases inaccessibility. The internal iliac vein system during lower anterior resections is a case in point. Aggressive dissection and electrocoagulation at the lateral border of the lesser pelvis can result in significant hemorrhage. Application of pressure is always preferable to electrocoagulation for the management of minor bleeding in the vicinity of major veins. In the event of major venous hemorrhage in this area, conversion and manual pressure are the first steps of management. Subsequently, if immediately available, consultation from a vascular surgeon should be obtained to explore all damage control options [17].

In the case of laparoscopic right colectomy for malignancy, the superior mesenteric vessels can be put under risk in the attempt to perform complete mesocolic excision. During attempts at identification of the middle colic vessels, injury may occur due to traction [18]. This avulsion type of injury can lead to damage of the main superior mesenteric vessels resulting in serious morbidity and mortality. Forceful manipulation of the mesocolon during the extra-corporeal phase of the procedure is another area of concern. The application of minimally invasive techniques does exclude the possibility of excessive application of force.

Anatomic variations in the distribution of vessels can also be an important factor leading to intraoperative bleeding [19]. In certain cases, such as that of the right gastric vessels, it should be noted that only a minority of individuals have a textbook distribution.

6.5   Bowel Injuries

Bowel injury is a serious complication because it can be missed at the time of the initial procedure. In open surgery, nonobvious bowel injuries can often be identified by the scent of enteral contents or the presence of enteral juice on laparotomy pads. This is not the case in laparoscopic surgery where, apart from the loss of tactile sense, there is a loss of olfactory sense.

Symptoms related to gastrointestinal injury usually appear during the second or third postoperative day but they can also manifest 5 or 7 days later [20].

Intestinal injuries during laparoscopy have been traditionally attributed to Veress needle or port placement or are caused by thermal injury from the electrocautery [21]. The small bowel is the most commonly injured organ but the colon can also be injured, especially when subcostal access techniques are used. Analyses from randomized controlled trials indicate that bowel injury is rare but is more frequently encountered in laparoscopic colorectal surgery (odds ratio 1.88) compared to open surgery [22]. In case of injury from insertion of the Veress needle, aspiration may show the presence of intestinal content. In that case, the needle should be retrieved, a new needle should be inserted in a different position, and the previous area should be carefully inspected. Intestinal injury can be repaired with 3–0 absorbable sutures.

Previous abdominal procedures and subsequent adhesions are a well-described risk factor for bowel injury. The separation of the adhesions is performed as close to the abdominal wall as possible so as not to injure any organs. Adhesions between viscera (e.g., between small bowel loops) can be more challenging. Conditions that are related to increased adhesion formation such as Crohn's disease and prior laparotomy are frequently cited as the major risk factors for conversion to open procedure [23]. In general, the use of sharp dissection is the preferred method. Liberal use of energy sources during this stage of the procedure can lead to inadvertent thermal injury that may not become apparent during the operation. Usually, there is a clearly defined avascular plane in the adhesions that renders the use of electrosurgery redundant in these cases. Minor bleeding adjacent to the surface of hollow viscera is preferable to aggressive use of electrocoagulation. In our experience, the application of pressure with the use of gauze is, in most cases, adequate for control of minor bleeding.

It should be noted that even in specialized centers, the incidence of small bowel injury is statistically greater in patients with a prior history of laparotomy than in patients without a history of open abdominal surgery [24]. Serosal abrasions or small enterotomies can be repaired primarily if the bowel segment has not been excessively damaged. Thermal injuries or larger-scale disruptions of enteral continuity will require an enterectomy and anastomosis.

6.6   Duodenal Injury

In contrast to open right colectomy, laparoscopic right colectomy is considered to be technically challenging due to difficulties in the identification of the proper plane. This is reflected in the longer operative times of laparoscopic right procedures compared to left procedures [25]. In most referral centers, a medial to lateral dissection is the preferred method, in which case the duodenum is recognized from a different point of view than in the open procedure. After ligation and division of the ileocolic vessels, the duodenum is recognized through an aperture created in the mesocolon. Meticulous dissection at the level of the duodenum and around the head of the pancreas should be upheld. It is of the upmost importance that dissection of the cecum and division of the posterior and medial attachments be continued up to the level of the duodenum. These steps are of paramount significance in order to avoid inadvertent injury to the duodenum. If injury is noted, the defect must be repaired laparoscopically or after a conversion to an open procedure, depending on the surgeon's preference and training. Unfortunately, inadvertent thermal injury can be difficult to discern during the procedure. Thermal injury may not be evident immediately and can manifest days after the completion of the procedure.

As it will be described later in this book, in the chapter discussing laparoscopic colectomy educational and training methods, the training of laparoscopic colectomy is a demanding process. This type of surgery has a steep learning curve requiring different, complementary training modalities for the surgeon to reach a desired level of skills and dexterity, especially in regards to the number of cases to be performed. Readers will have the opportunity to read more about education and best practices of laparoscopic colon surgery in a following chapter.

6.7   Ureter Injury

Ureteral injuries, in patients undergoing colorectal operations, have shown to be independently associated with higher mortality and morbidity. There is no clear consensus as to whether laparoscopic surgery is an independent risk factor for ureteral injury. A recent nationwide study in Denmark indicated that laparoscopic colorectal surgery for cancer with intent to cure was an independent risk factor for iatrogenic ureteral injury [26]. On the contrary, a retrospective study of procedures in the United States indicated that ureteral injuries were more common in open colectomies [27]. In some regards, this could be attributed to selection bias, as in the past 10–15 years open procedures have been reserved for locally aggressive tumors that make ureteral recognition more challenging. Regardless of which method is safer, the same safety precautions and the same risk factors apply to laparoscopic colectomy. Any factor which creates hostile local conditions such as reoperation, previous radiation therapy, large aggressive tumors, and tumor recurrence are all considered risk factors for iatrogenic[2] injury.

Iatrogenic injury occurs most often at the left ureter. The left ureter is in close proximity to the rectosigmoid colon in the region where it crosses over the left common iliac artery (Fig. 6.3). The ureter is mostly at risk when attempting to identify and ligate the superior rectal artery. Division of the lateral peritoneal attachments is

---

[2] Iatrogenic is the event that a physician or surgeon may cause inadvertently during medical treatment or medical diagnosis.

Fig. 6.3 Left
ureter anatomy

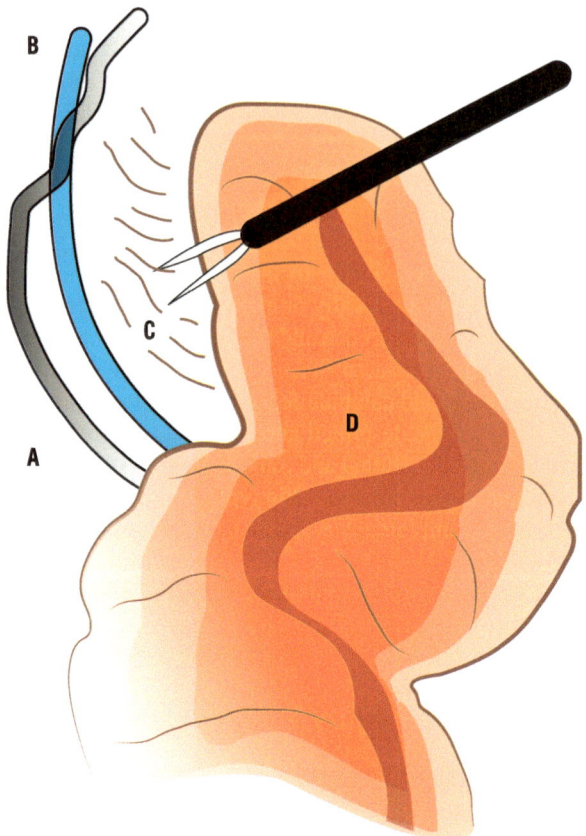

another step in the procedure where injury may occur. Undue medial traction of the sigmoid colon can alter the ureter's natural course. In that way, it can be mistaken for the superior mesenteric artery or another mesenteric vessel [28]. The right ureter is more vulnerable during the mobilization of the right colon by separating the ret-roperitoneal structures (ureter and gonadal vessels) from the terminal ileum and cecum (Fig. 6.4). This is performed by incising the virtually transparent peritoneal attachments of these structures laterally and rotating the cecum anteriorly and medi-ally. Injuries of the ureter can occur in several ways.

Approximately two-thirds of ureter injuries go unnoticed until symptoms become apparent postoperatively [29]. Most common injuries consist of complete transec-tion, suture ligation, excision of a segment or portion of the ureteral wall, heat dam-age from electrocautery, or devascularization. One-third of the injuries involve the distal ureter. These are primarily repaired with stent placement and ureteroneocys-tostomy. In greater loss of distal ureter length, a vesicopsoas hitch can be done. Upper and midureteral injuries are usually repaired by ureter anastomosis over an internal stent and in more significant loss of length a nephrostomy is indicated. The role of prophylactic stenting is still debated. Placement of a prophylactic stent may

Fig. 6.4 Right
ureter anatomy

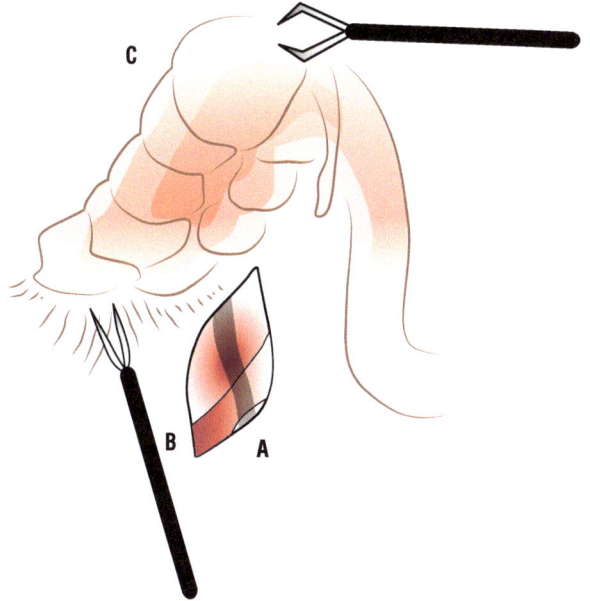

render identification easier but that does not necessarily correlate with fewer injuries [30]. Concerns regarding injury during placement and postoperative complications such as obstruction have limited the use in only selected cases such as bulky
tumors [31]. It has to be stressed that intraoperative identification is a prerequisite
but not a guarantee against injury.

6.8   Splenic Injury

Splenic injury seems to be less common in laparoscopic colorectal surgery compared to open surgery (odds ratio 6.58) because the visualization is better and forceful retraction is less [32]. When it happens, though, it most commonly occurs owing
to inadequate exposure and excess traction on the colon during mobilization of the
splenic flexure. Most injuries result from a capsular tear with avulsion of a small
segment of the splenic pulp. Attempt to control bleeding should begin with packing.
Topical hemostatic agents can be used. Other techniques as splenorrhaphy, the use
of omentum, and the use of topical hemostatic agents combined with a mesh wrap
have been described [33]. Splenic salvage is preferred, but splenectomy is usually
performed in case of uncontrollable bleeding. Based on findings from a large retrospective study from the Mayo clinic, the vast majority of splenic injuries (approximately 75%) were managed with a splenectomy [33]. It should be noted however
that this number included splenic injuries sustained during laparoscopic and open
surgery.

6.9   Failure in Lesion Localization

Small intraluminal tumors or endoscopically removed lesions can be impossible to localize even in open colorectal surgery. With the obvious loss of tactile sense in laparoscopic surgery, this is a more pressing problem. There are several reports that have documented the missing of small lesions after a laparoscopic colectomy [34]. Preoperative localization is an attractive modality. The placement of endoscopic clips or lesion tattooing has garnered the most attention. In the case of endoscopic clips, radiographic or ultrasonographic confirmation is usually employed [35]. Intraoperative colonoscopy is also an accepted option. A major concern in the use of endoscopic clips is the duration that they stay attached to the colonic mucosa. Clips can become dislodged at any moment and migrate to other portions of the colon.

Preoperative tattooing is another popular option. Timing is of crucial importance when contemplating the use of dyes for marking a lesion. Several dyes have been used such as methylene blue, isosulfan blue, indigo carmine, indocyanine green, and India ink.[3] With the exception of India ink, all these commercially available markers only have transient effects [36]. For example, in the case of methylene blue the effect has a duration of less than 24 h. Therefore, timing of tattooing is of particular importance. In our experience, with methylene blue, undue delays between tattooing and the procedure lead to diffusion of the dye along the serosa, which creates problems in the exact localization of the lesion. In addition, there needs to be standardization of the technique. Too little or too much dye can result in ambiguous results.

Despite these technical considerations, preoperative localization is invaluable to successful lesion localization and we routinely employ preoperative tattooing and use of clips in small size lesions. We use both techniques as a fail-safe in case tattooing yields ambiguous results due to diffusion. In the event that tattooing yields ambiguous results, we opt for intraoperative colonoscopy to identify the clips and guide resection.

6.10   Conversion to Open Surgery

Conversion to an open procedure is a likelihood during any laparoscopic procedure and every laparoscopic surgeon should be prepared for this event. Describing conversion to open surgery as a complication is technically a misnomer. However, inability to complete a procedure laparoscopically is frequently viewed as a "failure" on the part of the surgeon and for this reason we included conversion in our discussion of complications. In the opposite, when conditions dictate it, it indicates good surgical judgment. The reasons for converting to an open procedure include

---

[3] India ink or also known as Chinese ink is a black or colored ink that in the past had been used extensively for writing. Today it has medical applications and is also used for drawing and outlining.

unclear anatomy, excessive operative time, and intraoperative complications such as hemorrhage or organ injury. Most studies have documented that patients who have their operations converted have more frequent complications, longer postoperative hospital stays, and consequently higher costs [37]. Conversion rates vary greatly depending on pathology and surgeon's experience. In the case of malignancy, conversion rates vary from approximately 10–25% [37, 38]. Interestingly, the type of procedure seems to be an important factor in conversion rates. Transverse and left colectomies have been more likely to convert to open procedure (approximately 20%) [39, 40]. Other important independent factors are the presence of inflammation (e.g., diverticulitis, inflammatory bowel disease) and metastatic disease. When taking all pathologies into consideration, conversion rates have been reported up to 38% [40].

In a controlled study of 143 laparoscopic colectomies that were performed by the same, experienced surgeon in a period of 7 years (1993–2003), it was found that only 19.6% of cases have been converted to open surgery [41]. The experience of the surgeon can play a significant role in the conversion rate. According to the same study, conversion is considered a complication especially after considering that those cases that were converted showed higher postoperative wound complications, and greater length of stay [41], factors that increase the cost burden in a healthcare system and compromise the quality of care patients receive. To decrease the rate of conversion hand-assisted laparoscopic surgery (HALS) is recommended, especially in the case of obese patients whereas the working space becomes narrower and more difficult [42]. HALS may refrain a high-risk group of patients from conversion, saving them from the adverse effects related to conversion such as longer operative time, more blood loss, lengthier in-hospital stay, higher morbidity rate, and higher rates of reoperation and readmission [35]. To avoid complications and minimize morbidity, if a conversion is to be decided, this is better to be done in less than the first half hour of the operation because this time has been associated with fewer complications either intraoperative or postoperative [34, 35]. Extra efforts from the surgeon to complete the operation laparoscopically are shown to have more negative than positive results on the patient.

Special consideration should be given to locally aggressive tumors. If adjacent organs are involved such as duodenum, omentum, small bowel, ureter, or gonadal vessels, an en bloc[4] resection should be attempted. Aggressive dissection of the tumor that leads to malignant cell dispersal, inability to dissect, and ligate the appropriate lymphovascular pedicles should be avoided at all costs and conversion should be considered if this cannot be achieved laparoscopically. Conversion to open procedure does not seem to negatively affect oncological outcomes compared to upfront open colorectal surgery [38]. Nevertheless, careful patient selection and advanced surgical skills are the most important factors for a successful laparoscopic surgery. Careful preoperative evaluation as discussed in Chap. 4 of this book is crucial. Also, big, intensive training programs are required for surgeons to acquire the necessary

---

[4] *en bloc* resection is a term in oncology surgery referring to the resection of a large, bulky tumor without dissection.

skills to perform such demanding operations. Considering the limiting training hours, the cost of high in-operating-room training, and the changes in residents' curricula, alternative methods of training like the training on simulators can help surgeons develop the required skills to perform laparoscopic colon surgery in an effective way that would yield less morbidity, less days of hospitalization [43], and lower conversion rate.

6.11 Anastomotic Leak

A leak after colon anastomosis contributes a large amount of morbidity to the postoperative course. In colorectal surgery, anastomotic leaks are typically clinically evident after the fifth postoperative day although in certain cases they become clinically apparent after patient discharge [44].

Many local and systemic factors are believed to contribute to an increased rate of anastomotic leak. The two most important factors are the inadequate blood supply to the site of anastomosis and the presence of tension on the anastomosis. Failure in lesion localization the anastomosis (intraperitoneal or extraperitoneal) influences symptoms and therefore leaks may manifest with symptoms of generalized peritonitis, as a localized collection found on fever work-up or as a subclinical collection found on a contrast study. Predictive symptoms and signs include fever and leucocytosis, slow or no return of bowel function, increasing or suspicious drain output, oliguria, and renal failure. Randomized controlled trials have failed to show a significant difference between laparoscopic and open surgery in anastomotic leak prevention [45, 46]. They are both considered equally safe for the patient.

Clinical suspicion of a leak justifies reoperation. If inspection of the anastomosis reveals a defect in the staple line, reinforcing sutures can be placed. Unfortunately, in most cases, a diverting ostomy is unavoidable. Occasionally, a subclinical leak can be treated expectantly or with a percutaneous drainage procedure, under CT guidance.

Controversy persists over the choice of an intra-abdominal or extra-abdominal anastomosis. Meta-analysis has consistently failed to document a significant difference in anastomotic leak rates between these two types of anastomosis [47]. In the case of extra-abdominal anastomosis, special care needs to be taken to avoid excessive traction on the vascular pedicles as well to avoid unnecessary injury that could eventually compromise the blood supply. Therefore, we strongly recommend the implementation of the aforementioned principles of a well-vascularized anastomosis and avoidance of undue tension as a precaution against this complication.

6.12 Port Site Hernia

Initially, the closure of port sites after laparoscopic operations was vaguely addressed. Fascial closure was recommended only at the umbilical port site because the abdominal wall muscles were believed to prevent incisional hernias at the lateral port sites. However, many midline- as well as lateral-port site hernias have been reported. The clinical presentation varies from an asymptomatic lump at the port site to an acute incarcerated hernia with intestinal obstruction requiring emergency surgery. Size of the port (>12 mm), cutting trocars, and prolonged duration of the procedure have all been implicated in port site hernia formation [48].

An interesting variant of the port site hernia is the extraction site hernia. In cases of bulky specimens, a surgeon may opt to extend a preexisting incision to accommodate for the large specimen size. In our experience, we prefer to use the Pfannenstiel approach[5] and this is corroborated by data suggesting that hernia formation rate is relatively low in this position compared to midline extraction sites (3.8% vs 8.9%) [49].

6.13 Tumor Recurrence

One of the major, initial concerns regarding laparoscopic management of colon cancer was whether oncological outcomes would be comparable to the traditional open approach. During the past decade, large-scale randomized clinical trials addressed this issue. Laparoscopic colectomy demonstrates similar short-term and long-term oncological outcomes compared to an open approach [1, 50, 51]. There are no statistically significant differences in resection margins or lymph node dissection. Distribution of tumor recurrence sites (e.g., wound and port site recurrence or local recurrence) was also similar [1]. Based on these studies, laparoscopic colectomy is considered to be an equally acceptable option in regard to oncological outcomes.

However, in cases of rectal cancer, the data is inconclusive and recent studies indicate that oncological outcomes are inferior in non-Stage I cancer when laparoscopic techniques are employed [52]. This was demonstrated in a separate clinical trial even in cases of T1 tumors, indicating that laparoscopic approach is oncologically inferior [53]. A recent meta-analysis including trials over the past two decades demonstrated that laparoscopic rectal resection is associated with higher rates of incomplete total mesorectal excision, which is a key factor in rectal cancer recurrence [54]. Therefore, the literature suggests that at this point laparoscopic rectal cancer resection is not indicated in most cases.

6.14 Medical Complications

Deep venous thrombosis (DVT) is a major concern in major abdominal surgery, especially in the surgical treatment of colorectal cancer. Open abdominal surgery and malignancy are associated with a pro-inflammatory state in the recovery period and this can induce a thrombotic state. Delayed patient mobilization can lead to venous stasis in the extremities, which further increases the likelihood of

---

[5] Pfannenstiel approach is a pubic, abdominal surgical incision.

DVT. Retrospective data from the United States of America National Surgical Quality Improvement Program (NSQIP) suggests that DVT is significantly less common in laparoscopic partial colectomies (1.2% vs 0.003%) [6]. This difference did not seem to statistically influence mortality between the two groups. In addition, this benefit seems to extend in the elderly population as well as when examining partial colectomies [55].

Respiratory complications such as postoperative pneumonia are also a potential medical complication following major surgery that requires general anesthesia and endotracheal intubation. The aforementioned NSQIP data demonstrate that laparoscopic partial colectomies are associated with fewer respiratory complications including pneumonia. This may be attributed to better pain tolerance that results in better respiratory movement in the postoperative setting and/or earlier patient mobilization which limits postoperative atelectasis. There are questions regarding patients with preexisting respiratory conditions such as chronic obstructive pulmonary disease (COPD). Pneumoperitoneum can result in excessive atelectasis, which may not be well tolerated in this subset of patients. In the past, COPD was considered a relative contraindication in long laparoscopic procedures. There does not seem to be any recent evidence supporting this claim, and on the contrary laparoscopic colectomy is associated with fewer respiratory complications in these patients [56].

Other postoperative complications can be superficial or deep surgical site infections, dehiscence, pneumonia, pulmonary embolism, renal insufficiency, sepsis, septic shock, need for reintubation, ventilator failure, coma and cardiac arrest, bleeding, transfusions, urinary tract infection, and cerebral vascular accident. A 5-year retrospective cohort study found that laparoscopic colectomy is associated with lower rate of mortality and postoperative complications compared to open colectomy [57]. The surgeon's experience plays an important role in the improvement and the quality of the laparoscopic results.

6.15   Conclusions

Laparoscopic colorectal surgery is a safe alternative to open colorectal surgery, although it requires a long learning curve. As experience with these operative techniques has grown, rates of serious complications have become comparable and in most cases better than the results of the conventional operative approaches. Questions still remain unanswered in the management of rectal cancer. Inferior oncological outcomes render its application in this precarious setting. In certain cases, which are becoming less common with experience and continuous training, the management of intraoperative complications may require the conversion of the laparoscopic procedure to an open procedure. Therefore, the surgeon needs to be well versed in traditional operative techniques in order to ensure a safe surgical outcome in the most challenging cases.

Operative and postoperative outcomes of laparoscopic colectomy improve with time and experience. Adherence to continuous learning and training as well as careful selection and evaluation of patients contribute to the constant improvement of the technique's results, which lead to less complications, fewer days of hospitalization, and lower cost of treatment.

References

1. Fleshman J, Sargent DJ, Green E, et al. Laparoscopic colectomy for cancer is not inferior to open surgery based on 5-year data from the COST study group trial. Ann Surg. 2007;246:655–62; discussion 62-4
2. Bagshaw PF, Allardyce RA, Frampton CM, et al. Long- term outcomes of the Australasian randomized clinical trial comparing laparoscopic and conventional open surgical treatments for colon cancer: the Australasian laparoscopic colon cancer study trial. Ann Surg. 2012;256:915–9.
3. Schlachta CM, Mamazza J, Seshadri PA, Cadeddu M, Gregoire R, Poulin EC. Defining a learning curve for laparoscopic colorectal resections. Dis Colon Rectum. 2001;44:217–22.
4. Chen W, Sailhamer E, Berger DL, Rattner DW. Operative time is a poor surrogate for the learning curve in laparoscopic colorectal surgery. Surg Endosc. 2007;21:238–43.
5. Masoomi H, Kang CY, Chaudhry O, et al. Predictive factors of early bowel obstruction in colon and rectal surgery: data from the Nationwide inpatient sample, 2006-2008. J Am Coll Surg. 2012;214:831–7.
6. Wilson MZ, Hollenbeak CS, Stewart DB. Laparoscopic colectomy is associated with a lower incidence of postoperative complications than open colectomy: a propensity score-matched cohort analysis. Colorectal Dis. 2014;16:382–9.
7. Bailey MB, Davenport DL, Vargas HD, Evers BM, McKenzie SP. Longer operative time: deterioration of clinical outcomes of laparoscopic colectomy versus open colectomy. Dis Colon Rectum. 2014;57:616–22.
8. Ahmad G, Gent D, Henderson D, O'Flynn H, Phillips K, Watson A. Laparoscopic entry techniques. Cochrane Database Syst Rev. 2015;8:CD006583.
9. Dixon M, Carrillo EH. Iliac vascular injuries during elective laparoscopic surgery. Surg Endosc. 1999;13:1230–3.
10. la Chapelle CF, Swank HA, Wessels ME, Mol BW, Rubinstein SM, Jansen FW. Trocar types in laparoscopy. Cochrane Database Syst Rev. 2015;(12):CD009814.
11. Ott DE. Subcutaneous emphysema--beyond the pneumoperitoneum. JSLS. 2014;18:1–7.
12. Kamine TH, Elmadhun NY, Kasper EM, Papavassiliou E, Schneider BE. Abdominal insufflation for laparoscopy increases intracranial and intrathoracic pressure in human subjects. Surg Endosc. 2016;30:4029–32.
13. Kamine TH, Papavassiliou E, Schneider BE. Effect of abdominal insufflation for laparoscopy on intracranial pressure. JAMA Surg. 2014;149:380–2.
14. Epstein J, Arora A, Ellis H. Surface anatomy of the inferior epigastric artery in relation to laparoscopic injury. Clin Anat. 2004;17:400–8.
15. Mechchat A, Bagan P. Management of major vascular complications of laparoscopic surgery. J Visc Surg. 2010;147:e145–53.
16. Jafari MD, Pigazzi A. Techniques for laparoscopic repair of major intraoperative vascular injury: case reports and review of literature. Surg Endosc. 2013;27:3021–7.
17. Oderich GS, Panneton JM, Hofer J, et al. Iatrogenic operative injuries of abdominal and pelvic veins: a potentially lethal complication. J Vasc Surg. 2004;39:931–6.
18. Freund MR, Edden Y, Reissman P, Dagan A. Iatrogenic superior mesenteric vein injury: the perils of high ligation. Int J Color Dis. 2016;31:1649–51.
19. Lee SJ, Park SC, Kim MJ, Sohn DK, Oh JH. Vascular anatomy in laparoscopic colectomy for right colon cancer. Dis Colon Rectum. 2016;59:718–24.
20. Cassaro S. Delayed manifestations of laparoscopic bowel injury. Am Surg. 2015;81:478–82.

21. van der Voort M, Heijnsdijk EA, Gouma DJ. Bowel injury as a complication of laparoscopy. Br J Surg. 2004;91:1253–8.
22. Sammour T, Kahokehr A, Srinivasa S, Bissett IP, Hill AG. Laparoscopic colorectal surgery is associated with a higher intraoperative complication rate than open surgery. Ann Surg. 2011;253:35–43.
23. Masoomi H, Moghadamyeghaneh Z, Mills S, Carmichael JC, Pigazzi A, Stamos MJ. Risk factors for conversion of laparoscopic colorectal surgery to open surgery: does conversion worsen outcome? World J Surg. 2015;39:1240–7.
24. Yamamoto M, Okuda J, Tanaka K, et al. Effect of previous abdominal surgery on outcomes following laparoscopic colorectal surgery. Dis Colon Rectum. 2013;56:336–42.
25. Campana JP, Pellegrini PA, Rossi GL, Ojea Quintana G, Mentz RE, Vaccaro CA. Right versus left laparoscopic colectomy for colon cancer: does side make any difference? Int J Color Dis. 2017;32:907–12.
26. Andersen P, Andersen LM, Iversen LH. Iatrogenic ureteral injury in colorectal cancer surgery: a nationwide study comparing laparoscopic and open approaches. Surg Endosc. 2015;29:1406–12.
27. Halabi WJ, Jafari MD, Nguyen VQ, et al. Ureteral injuries in colorectal surgery: an analysis of trends, outcomes, and risk factors over a 10-year period in the United States. Dis Colon Rectum. 2014;57:179–86.
28. Nfonsam V, Aziz H, Pandit V, Khalil M, Jandova J, Joseph B. Analyzing clinical outcomes in laparoscopic right vs. left colectomy in colon cancer patients using the NSQIP database. Cancer Treat Commun. 2016;8:1–4.
29. Selzman AA, Spirnak JP. Iatrogenic ureteral injuries: a 20-year experience in treating 165 injuries. J Urol. 1996;155:878–81.
30. Bothwell WN, Bleicher RJ, Dent TL. Prophylactic ureteral catheterization in colon surgery. A five-year review. Dis Colon Rectum. 1994;37:330–4.
31. da Silva G, Boutros M, Wexner SD. Role of prophylactic ureteric stents in colorectal surgery. Asian J Endosc Surg. 2012;5:105–10.
32. Isik O, Aytac E, Ashburn J, et al. Does laparoscopy reduce splenic injuries during colorectal resections? An assessment from the ACS-NSQIP database. Surg Endosc. 2015;29:1039–44.
33. Holubar SD, Wang JK, Wolff BG, et al. Splenic salvage after intraoperative splenic injury during colectomy. Arch Surg. 2009;144:1040–5.
34. Stanciu C, Trifan A, Khder SA. Accuracy of colonoscopy in localizing colonic cancer. Rev Med Chir Soc Med Nat Iasi. 2007;111:39–43.
35. Montorsi M, Opocher E, Santambrogio R, et al. Original technique for small colorectal tumor localization during laparoscopic surgery. Dis Colon Rectum. 1999;42:819–22.
36. Hammond DC, Lane FR, Welk RA, Madura MJ, Borreson DK, Passinault WJ. Endoscopic tattooing of the colon. An experimental study. Am Surg. 1989;55:457–61.
37. Jayne DG, Thorpe HC, Copeland J, Quirke P, Brown JM, Guillou PJ. Five-year follow-up of the Medical Research Council CLASICC trial of laparoscopically assisted versus open surgery for colorectal cancer. Br J Surg. 2010;97:1638–45.
38. Yerokun BA, Adam MA, Sun Z, et al. Does conversion in laparoscopic colectomy portend an inferior oncologic outcome? Results from 104,400 patients. J Gastrointest Surg. 2016;20:1042–8.
39. Simorov A, Shaligram A, Shostrom V, Boilesen E, Thompson J, Oleynikov D. Laparoscopic colon resection trends in utilization and rate of conversion to open procedure: a national database review of academic medical centers. Ann Surg. 2012;256:462–8.
40. Lu KC, Cone MM, Diggs BS, Rea JD, Herzig DO. Laparoscopic converted to open colectomy: predictors and outcomes from the Nationwide inpatient sample. Am J Surg. 2011;201:634–9.
41. Belizon A, Sardinha CT, Sher ME. Converted laparoscopic colectomy. Surg Endosc. 2006;20(6):947–51. https://doi.org/10.1007/s00464-005-0553-3.
42. Heneghan HM, Martin ST, Kiran RP, Khoury W, Stocchi L, Remzi FH, Vogel JD. Laparoscopic colorectal surgery for obese patients: decreased conversions with the hand-assisted technique. J Gastrointest Surg. 2013;17(3):548–54. https://doi.org/10.1007/s11605-012-2089-x.

43. Matsiota E. Laparoscopic colectomy training: a quasi-experimental comparison of simulators to traditional training (order no. 3714872). Available from Dissertations & Theses @ University of Phoenix; ProQuest Central; ProQuest Dissertations & Theses Global. (1706722295). 2015. https://search-proquest-com.contentproxy.phoenix.edu/docview/1706722295?accoun tid=35812.
44. Hyman N, Manchester TL, Osler T, Burns B, Cataldo PA. Anastomotic leaks after intestinal anastomosis: it's later than you think. Ann Surg. 2007;245:254–8.
45. Clinical Outcomes of Surgical Therapy Study Group, Nelson H, Sargent DJ, et al. A comparison of laparoscopically assisted and open colectomy for colon cancer. N Engl J Med. 2004;350:2050–9.
46. Guillou PJ, Quirke P, Thorpe H, et al. Short-term endpoints of conventional versus laparoscopic-assisted surgery in patients with colorectal cancer (MRC CLASICC trial): multicentre, randomised controlled trial. Lancet. 2005;365:1718–26.
47. Cirocchi R, Trastulli S, Farinella E, et al. Intracorporeal versus extracorporeal anastomosis during laparoscopic right hemicolectomy - systematic review and meta- analysis. Surg Oncol. 2013;22:1–13.
48. Swank HA, Mulder IM, la Chapelle CF, Reitsma JB, Lange JF, Bemelman WA. Systematic review of trocar-site hernia. Br J Surg. 2012;99:315–23.
49. Samia H, Lawrence J, Nobel T, Stein S, Champagne BJ, Delaney CP. Extraction site location and incisional hernias after laparoscopic colorectal surgery: should we be avoiding the midline? Am J Surg. 2013;205:264–7; discussion 8
50. Lacy AM, Delgado S, Castells A, et al. The long-term results of a randomized clinical trial of laparoscopy- assisted versus open surgery for colon cancer. Ann Surg. 2008;248:1–7.
51. Colon Cancer Laparoscopic or Open Resection Study Group, Buunen M, Veldkamp R, et al. Survival after laparoscopic surgery versus open surgery for colon cancer: long-term outcome of a randomised clinical trial. Lancet Oncol. 2009;10:44–52.
52. Fleshman J, Branda M, Sargent DJ, et al. Effect of laparoscopic-assisted resection vs open resection of stage II or III rectal cancer on pathologic outcomes: the ACOSOG Z6051 randomized clinical trial. JAMA. 2015;314:1346–55.
53. Stevenson AR, Solomon MJ, Lumley JW, et al. Effect of laparoscopic-assisted resection vs open resection on pathological outcomes in rectal cancer: the ALaCaRT randomized clinical trial. JAMA. 2015;314:1356–63.
54. Martinez-Perez A, Carra MC, Brunetti F, de'Angelis N. Pathologic outcomes of laparoscopic vs open mesorectal excision for rectal cancer: a systematic review and meta-analysis. JAMA Surg. 2017;152:e165665.
55. Kannan U, Reddy VS, Mukerji AN, et al. Laparoscopic vs open partial colectomy in elderly patients: insights from the American College of Surgeons - National Surgical Quality Improvement Program database. World J Gastroenterol. 2015;21:12843–50.
56. Sujatha-Bhaskar S, Alizadeh RF, Inaba CS, et al. Respiratory complications after colonic procedures in chronic obstructive pulmonary disease: does laparoscopy offer a benefit? Surg Endosc. 2017;32(3):1280–5.
57. Wilson MZ, Dillon PW, Hollenbeak CS, Stewart B. How do risk factors for mortality and overall complication rates following laparoscopic and open colectomy differ between inpatient and post- discharge phases of care? A retrospective cohort study from NSQIP. Surg Endosc. 2014;28(12):3392–400. https://doi.org/10.1007/s00464-014-3609-4.

Robotic Colon Surgery and Quality of Life

A. Wilson Mourad and D. Daniel León

7.1 The Advent of Robotic Colon Surgery

The benefits for the patient of the minimally invasive surgical techniques have been supported through numerous studies. Nevertheless, the adoption of laparoscopic surgery in colon and rectum treatment remains limited. Even when large randomized controlled trials (e.g., COST in 2004 and COLOR II in 2013) have demonstrated the safety of laparoscopic approach in terms of oncologic outcomes, morbidity, and mortality rates, the colorectal surgery is still performed with the classic laparotomy by many surgeons. Compared to other complex surgical procedures such as bariatric or anti-reflux surgery, the adoption of minimally invasive techniques in colorectal procedures has followed a rather slow pace. In a study by Reanes et al. about the utilization rates of laparoscopic surgery in Medicare beneficiaries who underwent colon cancer resection surgery, it was found that, by 2010, only 32.5% of the resections were performed laparoscopically [1]. Other reports show similar rates of adoption of minimally invasive techniques for colorectal procedures. The National Institute for Health and Clinical Excellence (NICE) published their implementation uptake report of the percentage of colon and rectum resections performed with laparoscopy in England. According to their results, in 2007, only 8.8% of the procedures were performed with minimally invasive approach. This number increased to 22% in 2009 [2] but still until today the laparoscopic techniques are not the first preference for surgeons who perform colorectal surgery.

The main factors that restrain surgeons from employing the laparoscopic technique in colorectal surgery are the limited range of movement of the laparoscopic instruments, loss of three-dimensional views, and the lack of comprehensive

A. Wilson Mourad · D. Daniel León (✉)
CDD Las Mercedes, Caracas, Venezuela

© The Editor(s) (if applicable) and The Author(s),
under exclusive license to Springer Nature Switzerland AG 2021
G. Kouraklis, E. (J.) Matsiota (eds.), *Laparoscopic Colon Surgery*,
https://doi.org/10.1007/978-3-030-56728-6_7

training to perform complex laparoscopic surgical procedures. Robotic surgery could be a solution to some of these problems because it gives surgeons the options of motion scaling and augmented three-dimensional views with a stable camera and instruments that can imitate the range of motion of the human wrist. The first reports of robotic colectomies were published in 2002 by Weber et al., with one right and one left colectomy performed on benign tumors [3]. Since then, many authors have reported the feasibility of the use of the robotic platform for these procedures. Only 2 years later, D´Annibale et al. published a consecutive series of 106 colorectal procedures performed between 2001 and 2003. The da Vinci (Intuitive Surgical, Sunnyvale, CA, USA) robot was used in 53 patients for surgical treatment of colorectal diseases, and the outcomes were compared with the same number of patients who were surgically treated with conventional laparoscopy in the same period. In this first report, the researchers found no statistically significant difference between the laparoscopic and the robotic group in variables such as length of the specimen, number of lymphatic nodes harvested, recovery of bowel function, and length of hospital stay; meaning that the clinical outcomes for both procedures were equivalent. They noticed that the time required for the preparation of the operating room and the patient was significantly longer for the robotic group (24 ± 12 min) compared to the time registered for the laparoscopic group (18 ± 7 min). The authors emphasized that the dexterity and three-dimensional view of the robotic platform were important advantages over conventional laparoscopy in critical stages of the colonic resection, such as dissection of the splenic flexure, identification of vascular and nervous pelvic plexus, and hand-sewn anastomosis [4].

In 2013, Eriksen et al. published a retrospective analysis about the application of the robotic technology on colorectal procedures in a Danish, high-volume hospital. More than 200 colorectal procedures were performed with robotic assistance, including right and left colectomies, abdominoperineal resection, rectopexy, stoma reversal, and palliative procedures. The retrospective analysis showed a conversion rate to open surgery of 9% and a 16% of postoperative complications, comparable to previously published results [5].

To this date, accurate statistics reporting the use of robotics for colorectal procedures is scarce. Davis et al. published, in 2014, an analysis from a database of more than 600 healthcare facilities across the USA and selected patients older than 18 years who had undergone any type of colectomy performed with minimally invasive techniques. Laparoscopic and robotic procedures registered in the period from 2009 until the second quarter of 2011 were compared. A total of 25,758 records from patients who had undergone laparoscopic cecectomy, right or left hemicolectomy were analyzed. The results found only 2% (n: 548) of the procedures were performed with robotic assistance during this period [6].

In an observational study, Schootman et al. evaluated trends in the adoption of robotic-assisted surgery among hospitals and patients with colorectal cancer. By assessing American Hospital Association surveys and Nationwide Inpatient Sample in the years 2010 and 2012, the author concluded that high-volume, teaching hospitals, located in metropolitan areas, with advanced imaging services are more likely to adopt robotic surgery. These hospitals with high volume of cases can afford the cost of acquisition of robotic devices and the replacement of the disposable instruments, also have the presence of robotic-certified surgeons in their staff. Only 1.3% of colorectal cancer operations were performed with robotic assistance between 2010 and 2012, but the number is increasing, especially for patients with rectal cancer treated with minimally invasive techniques (2010: 5.5%; 2012: 13.3%). The authors explain that when working in narrow spaces such as male pelvis during rectal resections, the benefits of the robotic technology compared to laparoscopy become more evident [7]. This study also reflects that the acquisition and implementation of robotic devices across hospitals in the United States has increased during years, and by 2012, robots are present in more than 25% of the healthcare facilities evaluated, suggesting that this technology is becoming more available.

7.2   Robotic Colon Surgery Procedures and Techniques

With the proven benefits of the minimally invasive techniques in abdominal surgeries, all patients with colorectal diseases who require surgical treatment should be offered a minimally invasive approach. Nevertheless, patients with conditions such as severe respiratory or heart diseases that cause intolerance to pneumoperitoneum, bowel dilatation, or severe intra-abdominal adhesions because of previous surgeries should not be considered as prospects for robotic techniques; in such cases, the risk of conversion to open surgery would be high. In our experience, we have noted that the presence of large bulky tumors (over 12 cm diameter), pelvic abscess in complicated diverticular disease, or severe tumor adhesions to the pelvis or the abdominal wall are intraoperative findings that incommode the dissection with robotic instruments. A careful selection of patients during presurgical evaluation is highly recommended to keep the conversion rate to laparoscopic or open surgery under 15%. Prior to surgery, the patient must be prepared with oral administered colon cleansers, rectal enemas, and oral intake of antibiotics, as is done with conventional laparoscopic elective colectomies. For more details about the preoperative selection of patients, the reader may refer to the chapter of Preoperative Evaluation and Selection of Patients in this book.

The robotic-assisted techniques use the robotic platform to perform a partial or total dissection depending on the extent of the disease. Conventional laparoscopy may be used in one part of the procedure. An extracorporeal anastomosis is performed with sutures or with staplers. Comprehensive robotic procedures use the robotic platform during the entire surgery, including an intracorporeal anastomosis, either with hand-sewn or with endostapler. The selection between a robotic-assisted or complete robotic procedure depends on factors such as the experience of the surgeon in intracorporeal suturing, the availability of resources such has the new da Vinci Xi (Intuitive Surgical Inc., Mountain View, CA, USA) platform with features that allow multi-quadrant surgery, and the thickness of the abdominal wall; a gross fat tissue limits the movements of the trocars and the reach of the instruments into the abdominal cavity.

7.2.1   Robotic Right Colectomy

A right colectomy involves the resection of the distal ileon, 10–15 cm before the ileocecal valve, the ascending colon, and the first third of the transverse colon, with a side-to-side ileocolic anastomosis and closure of the mesenteric space. In our practice, an 8-mm port is placed at the left side of the umbilicus for the camera and two 8-mm ports, for both robotic arms manipulated by the console surgeon, are placed 10 cm away from the camera in an arched-fashion line. A 12-mm trocar is placed on the left upper quadrant for irrigation/suction, for bowel traction, or to introduce an endostapler by the assistant (Fig. 7.1). The procedure itself follows the same steps as a laparoscopic right colectomy. A medial to lateral dissection can be performed; however, we routinely perform the dissection of the ascending colon with a lateral-to-medial and inferior-to-superior approach. The right ureter and gonadal vessels are identified and preserved, then identification and ligation of the ileocolic vessels, and separation of the colon and the hepatic flexure from the retroperitoneum follow. The first third of the transverse colon and its mesentery are carefully separated from the duodenum, and the right branch of the median colic artery is identified. Once the endpoints of resection are marked, the surgeon must decide either to perform an intracorporeal ileocolic anastomosis or to perform an abdominal incision next to the operation site to extract the specimen and to perform an extracorporeal ileocolic anastomosis. The 7-degree of movement of the robotic arms allows the surgeon to perform a sewn ileocolic anastomosis with no major

Fig. 7.1 Location of the trocars for a robotic right colectomy. The number inside the circles indicates the diameter of the trocar. C = Camera port (8 mm diameter)

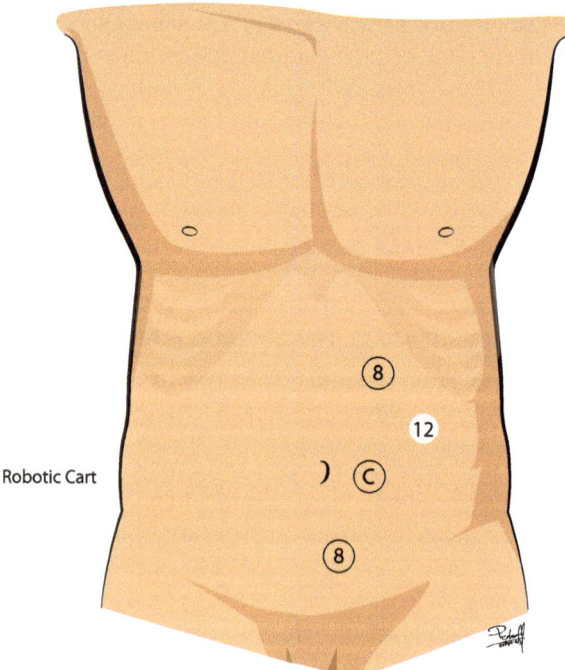

difficulties. Then, the specimen can be extracted through a Pfannenstiel[1] incision for better cosmetic results. An extracorporeal ileocolic anastomosis might be easier and faster to perform, but may leave a large visible scar over the abdominal wall. The decision of performing an intracorporeal or extracorporeal anastomosis in patients undergoing robotic right colectomy depends on the preferences and experience of the surgeon with laparoscopic suturing; the published data regarding advantages of one technique over the other are controversial. We recommend individualizing patients and in those with a short mesenterium or gross fat tissue, that might require larger incisions in the abdominal wall, to perform an intracorporeal anastomosis and specimen extraction through a suprapubic Pfannenstiel incision.

A review and meta-analysis published by Oostendorp et al. in 2017, comparing intracorporeal and extracorporeal anastomosis in right colectomy, found that the length of hospital stay and the morbidity are significantly lower when an intracorporeal anastomosis is performed (MD = 0.77 days, 95% CI −1.46 to −0.07 and OR 0.68, 95% CI 0.49–0.93, respectively). Mortality, ileus, and anastomotic leakage showed no difference between the two techniques [8]. In a meta-analysis published by Rondelli et al. (2015), the extracorporeal laparoscopic and intracorporeal robotic anastomosis were compared. The results showed no statistically significant differences in the incidence of anastomotic leakage, wound infections, or postoperative ileus between the two techniques. The length of hospital stay was found to be lower for the robotic group when an intracorporeal ileocolic anastomosis was performed [9].

Xu et al. (2014) compared robotic versus laparoscopic right colectomy through a meta-analysis that evaluated seven studies with a total of 649 patients, divided into two groups (234 in the robotic right colectomy group and 415 in the laparoscopic right colectomy group). This meta-analysis found a faster recovery of the bowel function in the robotic right colectomy group compared to the laparoscopic group. The advantages of the three-dimensional views and the multiple degree movement of the robotic instruments make it easier to perform an intracorporeal anastomosis. Other advantage observed with intra corporeal anastomosis was the significantly lower risk of incisional hernia because of the smaller incision needed for specimen extraction. No differences were found between groups concerning the anastomotic leakage or the postoperative bleeding [10].

Both meta-analysis studies of Rondelli et al. (2015) and Xu et al. (2014) showed significantly longer operating time for the robotic group compared to the laparoscopic group (Rondelli: MD = 54.36, 95% CI: 37.30–71.43; $p < 0.00001$; Xu: MD = 48.24; 95% CI: 28.82–67.66; $p < 0.00001$) and lower estimated blood loss in the robotic group, thus requiring no transfusions during surgery. No difference was observed in the length of hospital stay, the conversion rates to open surgery, the number of lymph nodes harvested, or the postoperative complications. The operating time for robotic right colectomy seems to be longer when compared with its laparoscopic counterpart. The results for the operating time in the robotic groups were longer compared with laparoscopic groups (MD = 48.24; 95% CI: 28.82–67.66;

---

[1] Pfannenstiel is a type of abdominal surgical incision that allows the surgeon to have access to the abdomen. It is mainly used in Caesarian sections.

$P < 0.00001$). The time required to prepare the robot before the surgery, and to undock it from the patient after the resection, consumes time in the operating room. The same studies have observed that the experience of the surgical team and the learning curve are influential factors in reducing long operating times [9, 10].

7.2.2 Robotic Left Colectomy

A left colectomy involves the resection of the second half of the transverse colon, the descending and sigmoid colon until the upper rectum, usually with an end-to-end double-stapled colorectal anastomosis. In some cases, a permanent colostomy may be necessary.

Contrary to the conventional laparoscopy, where the surgeon can move around the quadrants of the abdomen with no major restriction, the robotic cart, once it's docked, allows the surgeon a limited capacity to move from one quadrant to another. Thus, the mobilization of the splenic flexure is the main challenge during a left robotic colectomy. This issue has led to the development of three different techniques for multi-quadrant robotic procedures: (a) the single-docking totally robotic, (b) the double docking, and (c) the hybrid technique [11, 12].

7.2.2.1 The Single-Docking Technique

In our experience and in our practice with the da Vinci Xi (Intuitive Surgical Inc., Mountain View, CA, USA) platform, the mobilization of the splenic flexure can be achieved with a single-docking technique, thus allowing to perform a totally robotic left colectomy without changing trocars or redocking the patient's cart. The rotation of the boom in the patient's cart makes the docking process easier and, if needed, the process of undocking and redocking is faster and effortless. The trocar placement for totally robotic left colectomies is shown in Fig. 7.2. The suprapubic 8-mm trocar can be expanded for specimen retrieval.

There are no specific indications to choose between a totally robotic or a robotic-assisted left colectomy. Mégevand et al. (2016) have described their experience performing a single-docking technique for a totally robotic left colectomy, using the da Vinci Si (Intuitive Surgical, Sunnyvale, CA) system. The aim of this technique is to reduce the operating time by optimizing the trocar placement, thus avoiding conflict of the instruments or moving the patients' cart during the different stages of the procedure. Mégevand describes a trocar location similar to the one showed in Fig. 7.2, but the assistant uses a 12-mm port located in position "B," and the epigastric port is used for the robotic arm 2. The dissection follows a clockwise direction from medial to lateral, starting at the splenic flexure then descending to the rectum. Difficulties were present in cases of high insertion of the splenic flexure. In such case, the trocar of the robotic arm 1 must be introduced a few centimeters to allow the instrument to reach the anatomic target, thus modifying the fulcrum point of the trocar. As the descending dissection continues after ligation of the inferior mesenteric vein and artery, flipping instruments between robotic arms 2 and 3 may be necessary in order to avoid conflict during retraction of the rectum and dissection of pelvic fascia, and neurovascular plexus. This study included 83 consecutive cases of

Fig. 7.2 Schematic view of the trocar placement for double- or single-docking robotic left colectomy. The 8-mm port in the right upper quadrant (A) for the assistant can be switched to dock a robotic arm during dissection of the splenic flexure and used by the assistant during the pelvic dissection. C = Camera, A = Assistant, B and D are used for robotic arms during pelvic dissection. E = used during sigmoid dissection and extended for specimen retrieval

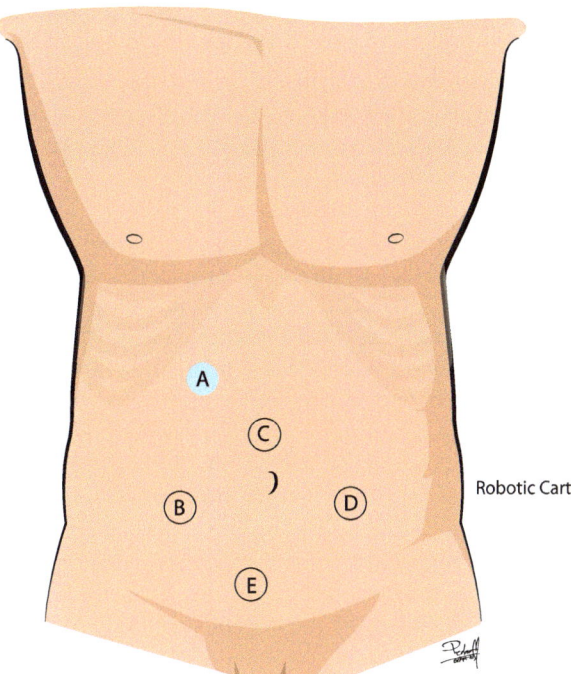

Robotic Cart

patients with sigmoid or middle-low rectal cancer between May 2012 and June 2016, all performed with single-docking technique without conversions to laparoscopic or open surgery. The authors stressed the important role of the assistant surgeon to prevent collisions and malfunctioning of the instruments during surgery. A decrease in the total operating time, as the surgical team gained experience, is mentioned in the study but not clearly specified [14].

7.2.2.2 The Double-Docking Technique

The double-docking technique for totally robotic left colectomy is useful when utilizing the former generations of the robotic platforms. This technique requires a first step of docking for the mobilization of the splenic flexure; then undocking, mobilization of the robotic cart, and redocking during surgery for dissection of the sigmoid and upper rectum in order to perform a totally robotic left colectomy. This technique might need extra robotic ports during the mobilization of the splenic flexure and later redocking of the robotic cart for dissection of the sigmoid colon and upper rectum. The process of changing trocars and docking several times during surgery increases the operative times [13].

7.2.2.3 The Hybrid Technique

The hybrid technique uses conventional laparoscopy for the mobilization of the splenic flexure, the descending colon, and the ligation of the left colic artery. Then, the robotic cart is docked to perform the dissection of the sigmoid colon, the upper rectum, and its mesentery. The hybrid technique has as advantages the use of only three working ports and does not require mobilization or redocking the robotic cart.

The hybrid technique is used to perform the mobilization of the splenic flexure with laparoscopic instruments and then the robot is used for dissection of the pelvic structures including lymphovascular dissection. The aim of this approach is to reduce the time necessary to undock, relocate, and redock the patients' cart. Patients with a high body mass index (BMI) or a tumor, deep located in pelvis, might benefit from this technique.

Park JE et al. (2016) have described a "reverse-hybrid" technique, where a robotic approach for the dissection of vascular and pelvic structures is performed as first step and then laparoscopy for splenic flexure mobilization follows. The patient is positioned in Trendelenburg[2] and lithotomy modified position, thus permitting to dock the robotic cart between the patient's legs. This location allows an optimal mechanical operation of the robotic arms in pelvic surgeries. The splenic flexure mobilization and inferior mesenteric vein dissection are laparoscopically performed; the operating table facilitates the repositioning to reverse Trendelenburg. Between January 2009 and March 2011, 30 patients with histologically confirmed rectal adenocarcinoma underwent surgical resection and the results of this technique were evaluated. The authors report no conversion to open surgery or intraoperative complications. The average operative time was 369 minutes (varying from 306 to 410 min) and the median time attributed to the use of the robotic console was 98 min (30.9% of the total operation time). One case of small bowel obstruction, one anastomotic leak, and one bleeding case from the inferior mesenteric artery were reported as postoperative complications. Obese patients or those who required extended or extramesorectal pelvic lymph node resection did not benefit from the minimally invasive approach before the introduction of the robotic surgery [15].

The robotic left colectomy has been feasible, safe, and offering clinical outcomes similar or better to the laparoscopic resections. Between 2006 and 2008 Lim et al. evaluated prospectively 180 patients with diagnosis of sigmoid adenocarcinoma who underwent either laparoscopic or robotic anterior resection (146 and 34 respectively). The assessment of demographic and clinical parameters such as patient age, sex, mean BMI, ASA[3] score, tumor location, and other results was comparable. In this study, the robotic anterior resection showed better clinical outcomes than the laparoscopic anterior resection. Some parameters, indicative of the clinical recovery after abdominal surgery, such as days to first flatus, stool passing, days to start diet, and days of hospitalization, were statistically lower in the robotic patients' group. The oncologic outcome after 3 years' follow-up showed similar results for both groups. The average operating time was longer for the robotic group: 252.5 ± 94.9 min (95% CI, 219.3–285.6 min) compared to the laparoscopic group 217.6 ± 70.7 min (95% confidence interval [CI], 205.6–229.1 min) ($p = 0.016$). Besides the time required to dock the patient's cart, the process of changing instruments during robotic procedures is time-consuming, thus increasing operating time compared to the laparoscopic procedure [16].

---

[2] For patient's and surgeon's positioning please refer to Fig. 4.1 of the Chap. 4 of this book.

[3] ASA is a subjective assessment of a patient's health. The assessment is based on five classes (I to V) of physical health as identified by the American Society of Anesthesiologists.

7.2.3 Robotic Rectal Surgery

The experience gained in the urological field with the use of the robotic technology has promoted its use to the colorectal surgeons' community for the surgical treatment of rectal diseases, such as cancer and rectal prolapse.

As with right- or left-side colectomy, the preparation of the patient before surgery is the same as for the conventional laparoscopic procedures. Colon cleansers and rectal enemas must be administered 24 h prior to surgery and oral antibiotics are indicated. For more information about the presurgical preparation of the patient, the reader should refer to the chapter Preoperative Evaluation and Selection of Patients of this book.

Pneumoperitoneum is insufflated and an 8-mm camera trocar is placed 3–4 cm upper from the umbilicus. The two 8-mm trocars for the robotic arms are inserted both the sides at a distance of 10 cm from the camera port. The fourth robotic arm can be placed on the left for traction purposes, and a 5-mm trocar for irrigation/suction and bowel traction by the assistant can be placed at the right (Fig. 7.3).

All rectal procedures such as low anterior resection, abdominoperineal resection, total mesorectal excision, or rectopexy are performed following the steps classically described. Urinary and sexual impairment symptoms have been reported after open or laparoscopic procedures that involve the rectum or other pelvic organs. These symptoms are caused by the manipulation of the autonomic nerves during procedures such as total mesorectal excision (TME).

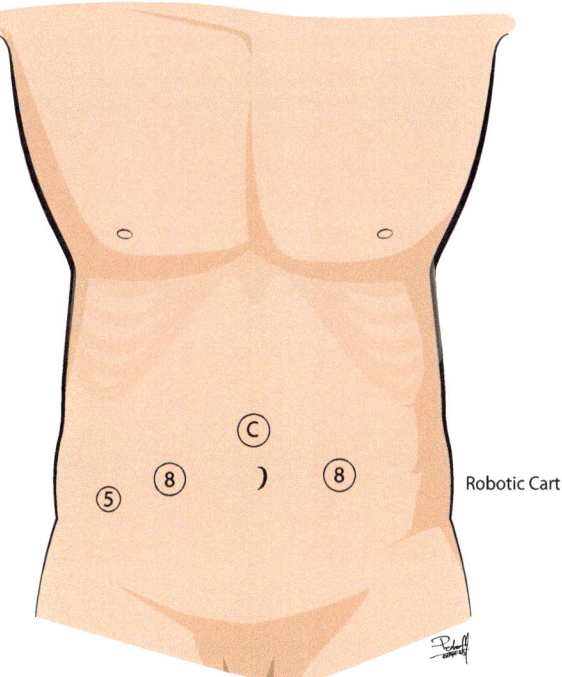

Fig. 7.3 Trocar placement for robotic rectal surgery. C = Camera, the number inside the circles indicates de diameter of the trocars

To evaluate if robotics offer advantages over laparoscopic techniques regarding urinary symptoms after rectal surgery, several authors have compared short- and long-term outcomes of robotic procedures performed over rectum. Panteleimonitis et al. [17] compared the urological and sexual functional outcomes of laparoscopic and robotic rectal cancer surgery in men and women. Using specific questionnaires for urological and sexual function, their study assessed components such as urinary frequency, nycturia, libido, orgasm, and dyspareunia, among others. Results of this study showed favorable changes for the robotic group from baseline in composite mean male urinary function (MUF) and also for mean composite scores of male sexual function (MSF). Compared to laparoscopy, the robotic group showed a worst outcome only in symptoms related to initiation/straining. On the other hand, women showed no statistical difference in any score of the female urological function (FUF) components from baseline between groups, with better postoperative scores after robotic surgery and worse after laparoscopic surgery. Regarding the female sexual function (FSF) both groups had similar results with no statistical difference between the mean change of scores from the baseline. However, the authors recognize that due to a small number of patients being sexually active, the sample was too small to make a meaningful statistical analysis.

In another study, Wang et al. [18] prospectively evaluated urinary and sexual function in male patients who underwent rectal cancer surgery. After applying the exclusion criteria, 137 patients were enrolled and randomly allocated into laparoscopic or robotic surgery procedures (66 and 71 respectively). Urinary and sexual functions were assessed in all patients preoperatively and 12 months postoperatively using International Prostate Symptom Score (IPSS) and International Index of Erectile Function (IIEF). Urinary function was assessed using IPSS and average time of catheter removal, observing that urethral decatheterization was significantly earlier in the robotic surgery group compared to the laparoscopic.

Most patients had urinary symptoms prior to surgery (mean IPSS score: 4.07), but postoperatively, the laparoscopic group showed a significant increase in IPSS scores (9.66 vs 4.12; $p = 0,031$). On the contrary, the robotic group showed no differences in pre and postoperative scores, in total IPSS scores, as well as in the evaluation of specific symptoms. When laparoscopic and robotic groups were compared, results of postoperatively IPSS scores were significantly lower in patients who underwent robotic compared to laparoscopic procedures (Table 7.1).

Male sexual function was pre and postoperatively evaluated with IIEF. Total postoperative IIEF scores were significantly lower for both groups compared to preoperative. When the laparoscopic groups were compared with the robotic groups, the total IIEF postoperative scores were higher in the later. The authors report a lower incidence of sexual dysfunction in patients after robotic procedures, compared with patients who underwent laparoscopic surgeries. Additional to these data, during the study, 10 postoperative complications were observed in the laparoscopic group and eight in the robotic group; a relationship between postoperative complications and final outcome was not reported.

By 2014, Broholm et al. [19] conducted a meta-analysis to evaluate results of studies reporting dysfunction of urinary and genital apparatus after robotic-assisted

Table 7.1 Urinary function before and after surgery

	Laparoscopic surgery (n = 66)			Robotic surgery (n = 71)		
	Pre-op	Postop	p	Pre-op	Postop	p
Total IPSS	4.12 ± 5.48	9.66 ± 5.74[a]	0.031	4.04 ± 5.26	5.79 ± 5.69[b]	0.061
Incomplete emptying	0.33 ± 0.67	0.97 ± 1.16	0.118	0.37 ± 0.79	0.81 ± 0.96	0.428
Frequency	0.54 ± 0.87	1.31 ± 1.71[a]	0.043	0.67 ± 0.96	1.01 ± 1.24	0.381
Intermittency	0.47 ± 0.91	1.14 ± 1.06	0.082	0.43 ± 0.84	0.73 ± 0.98[b]	0.152
Urgency	0.48 ± 0.67	0.91 ± 1.22	0.351	0.31 ± 0.73	0.84 ± 1.05	0.417
Weak stream	0.81 ± 1.21	1.86 ± 1.73	0.284	0.76 ± 1.24	1.04 ± 1.26[b]	0.158
Straining	0.66 ± 0.96	1.17 ± 1.14	0.117	0.61 ± 1.05	0.97 ± 1.17	0.331
Nocturia	0.97 ± 1.14	2.23 ± 2.05[a]	0.035	0.94 ± 1.27	1.44 ± 2.11	0.489

From: Wang G, Wang Z, Jiang Z, Liu J, Zhao J, Li J. Male urinary and sexual function after robotic -pelvic autonomic nerve-preserving surgery for rectal cancer. Int J Med Robotics Comput Assist Surg 2017; 13: 1
[a]p 0.05 for postoperative vs pre-operative values
[b]$p < 0.05$ for robotic vs laparoscopic operation

surgery in patients with rectal cancer. Through a systematic search in PubMed, Cochrane Library, and Embase databases, relevant articles published prior to February 2014 were selected. All reports were evaluated to detect risk of bias; the meta-analysis results were assessed based on the Grading of Recommendations, Assessments, Development and Evaluations (Grade) approaches. Regarding IPSS, authors found a statistically significant difference of IPSS scores in favor of robotic procedures after a 3-month follow-up (mean difference (MD) = 1.58, 95% confidence interval $(-3.1–0.05)$, $p = 0.04$). After 6 months follow-up, the pooled results showed no significant difference (MD = 0.59, 95% CI $(-2.00–0,82)$, $p = 0.41$), and after 12 months follow-up, the improvement on IPSS score after robotic surgery was statistically significant (MD = 0.90, 95% CI: $-1.81–0.02$), $p = 0.05$). When evaluating erectile function, three studies met the selection criteria for meta-analysis, with 128 patients at 3 and 125 patients at 6 months follow-up. During both periods, the pooled estimates showed better results after robot-assisted surgery than laparoscopic.

It is important to notice that the Grade approach used to assess the quality of the evidence resulted in a very low score. Hence, these outcomes were downgraded due to the design of the studies, high possibility of bias, and imprecise data. This meta-analysis showed that compared to laparoscopic surgery, robotic-assisted surgery for rectal cancer offers better outcomes in sexual function, and the urinary function seems to be improved, but results are not consistent and must be carefully interpreted as all studies available were nonrandomized and the population of patients included was small.

Benign conditions such as rectal prolapse have a negative impact on the quality of life of patients caused mainly by symptoms such as constipation, pelvic pain, and rectal bleeding. Currently, the abdominal approach is preferred over perineal surgery because of the higher recurrence rates of the latter.

Functional outcome of robotic ventral mesh rectopexy for rectal prolapse in different studies have shown no significant difference in results (obstructed defecation, residual prolapse, continence, and recurrence rates) compared to the laparoscopic ventral mesh rectopexy. There may be a trend towards a better outcome for obstructed defecation following robotic mesh rectopexy as compared to the laparoscopic procedure, but the level of evidence is low [20, 21].

7.3   Additional Benefits of the Robotic Surgery in the Quality of Life of Patients

The evaluation of quality of life in patients undergoing colorectal surgery must consider several parameters; besides urological and sexual outcomes mentioned above, the surgeon must evaluate the quality of life after surgery, particularly if a permanent stoma is created, or if a low anterior resection (LAR) is performed. Other considerations include postoperative pain, postoperative time to resume diet, and return to common daily activities.

The risk of anastomotic leaks after colorectal procedures remains one of the biggest challenges. Performing anastomosis in a viscera, with a high load of bacteria, represents a major problem when anastomotic leaks appear because they may lead to sepsis, and in many cases the need of a reintervention, resulting in a non-initially planned colostomy. Small leaks that do not require surgical intervention as first treatment may end up with strictures that decrease the lumen diameter or with bowel dysfunction that cause long-term discomfort on the affected patient and multiple consultations to the health centers to deal with chronic problems. Several interventions have been proposed to prevent or decrease the risk of anastomotic leaks. Evaluation of blood supply at the resection borders has traditionally been assessed intraoperatively by inspecting the color and bleeding of the bowel at the cutting ends. Recent techniques involve the intravenous administration of fluorophore substances to perform perfusion angiographies enabling the surgeon to assess tissue perfusion in real time [22, 23].

The da Vinci Xi (Intuitive Surgical Inc., Mountain View, CA, USA) robotic system has incorporated near-infrared reflectance (NIR) technology to its three-dimensional camera called FireFly TM [24]. The most commonly used fluorophore is FDA-approved indocyanine green (ICG), which when intravenously administered distributes in the intravascular space and after activation of NIR mode camera, the ICG is seen as white fluorescence in a black background, thus, demonstrating tissue blood perfusion. Kim et al. [23] evaluated the utility of perfusion angiography with indocyanine during sphincter-saving operation (SSO) robotically performed. Between the years 2010 and 2014, a consecutive cohort of 436 rectal cancer patients underwent robot-assisted SSO, including 123 patients with indocyanine green (ICG) imaging (ICG+ group). The anastomotic leaks reported rate for the ICG+ group was 0.8%, compared to 5.4% in the ICG− group ($p = 0.031$). These results are similar to the ones reported by other studies that evaluated fluorescence perfusion angiography with laparoscopic techniques.

Even when ICG angiography may not necessarily be routinely performed, the authors conclude that it enables safe anastomosis in individuals with a high risk of anastomotic site ischemia, such as patients with anatomical variations in the marginal and rectal vasculatures, or narrow left mesocolon. Fluorescence angiography using ICG is also a useful resource to help identify lymph nodes (due to its green fluorescence) in obese patients, thus allowing the surgeon to perform appropriate lymph node resection in rectal cancer patients for optimal oncological outcomes.

7.4 Conclusions

The adoption of robotic surgery for colorectal procedures has increased along years; the number of robotic procedures is increasing mostly in teaching hospitals and metropolitan areas, with major acceptance for procedures involving the rectum. Despite the advancements in medical knowledge and in new technologies, colorectal surgery remains challenging in terms of short- and long-term outcomes, complications, and functional results. Several interventions have been made to solve different problems of colorectal surgery and implementation of new technologies is always present. To this date, the use of robotic platform in colorectal surgery has demonstrated to be feasible and safe for the patient, with equivalent outcomes to laparoscopy in terms of oncologic and pathological results. Many studies have found benefits in the use of robotics in colorectal procedures, such as reduction of rate of complications, fewer cases of anastomotic leakage, and fewer days of hospital stay, among others.

The right colectomy for malignant or benign diseases, with either intra or extracorporeal anastomosis, is feasible and safe to be performed with robotic techniques, with drawbacks in prolonged operative time, mostly attributable to the process of docking the patient's cart and to the steep learning curve. Left colectomies can be performed with robotic devices, but the limited range of movement of the robotic cart, once docked to the patient, is a problem that needs to be solved in order to standardize the technique for totally robotic procedure.

As with laparoscopy when it was first introduced, longer operative times and higher costs are seen with robotic surgeries. Operative time has proven to reduce with surgical team's increased experience. Because the acquisition of robotic platforms is expensive as is its maintenance cost, the robotic surgery is still far from being massively applied. The generalization of technologies and the broader use and wider acceptance of robotics in colon surgery can increase the usage rate and reduce the cost, while improving the efficiency of the resources. The long-term outcomes of rectal robotic surgeries are promising in preserving sexual and urological function, but these results must be carefully considered because of a small number of cases included in the studies and the high possibility of bias.

Robotic surgery is becoming more widely present, thus benefiting more patients undergoing surgery with minimally invasive techniques. Randomized controlled trials with larger populations and longer follow-up periods such as the ROLARR study (Robotic versus Laparoscopic Resection for Rectal Cancer) are ongoing and its results will bring more light on current concerns.

References

1. Reames BN, Sheetz KH, Waits SA, Dimick JB, Regenbogen SE. Geographic variation in use of laparoscopic colectomy for colon cancer. J Clin Oncol. 2014;32(32):3667–72. https://doi.org/10.1200/JCO.2014.57.1588.
2. Pascual M, Salvans S, Pera M. Laparoscopic colorectal surgery: current status and implementation of the latest technological innovations. World J Gastroenterol. 2016;22(2):704–17. https://doi.org/10.3748/wjg.v22.i2.704.
3. Weber PA, et al. Telerobotic-assisted laparoscopic right and sigmoid colectomies for benign disease. Dis Colon Rectum. 2002;45(12):1689–94; discussion 1695-6
4. D'Annibale A, et al. Robotic and laparoscopic surgery for treatment of colorectal diseases. Dis Colon Rectum. 2004;47(12):2162–8.
5. Eriksen JR, et al. Early results after robot-assisted colorectal surgery. Dan Med J. 2013;60(12):A4736.
6. Davis B, Yoo A, et al. Robotic-assisted versus laparoscopic colectomy: cost and clinical outcomes. JSLS. 2014;12:211–4.
7. Schootman M, et al. Adoption of robotic Technology for Treating Colorectal Cancer. Dis Colon Rectum. 2016;59(11):1011–8.

8. Van Oostendorp S, Elfrink A, Borstlap W, et al. Intracorporeal versus extracorporeal anastomosis in right hemicolectomy: a systematic review and meta- analysis. Surg Endosc. 2017;31(1):64–77. https://doi.org/10.1007/s00464-016-4982-y.
9. Rondelli B, et al. Is robot-assisted right colectomy more effective than the conventional laparoscopic procedure? A meta-analysis of short term outcomes. Int J Surg. 2015;18:75–82.
10. Xu H, et al. Robotic versus laparoscopic right colectomy: a meta-analysis. World J Surg Oncol. 2014;12:274.
11. Park EJ, Baik SH. Robotic surgery for colon and rectal cancer. Curr Oncol Rep. 2016;18:5. https://doi.org/10.1007/s11912-0150491-8.
12. Isik O, Gorgun E. How has the robot contributed to colon cancer surgery? Clin Colon Rectal Surg. 2015;28(4):220–7. https://doi.org/10.1055/s-0035-1564436.
13. Kim CW, Kim CH, Baik SH. Outcomes of robotic-assisted colorectal surgery compared with laparoscopic and open surgery: a systematic review. J Gastrointest Surg. 2014;18(4):816–30. https://doi.org/10.1007/s11605-014-2469-5.
14. Mégevand J, Rusconi A, Amboldi M, Lillo L, Lenisa L, et al. Totally robotic low anterior resection and left colectomy with systematic splenic flexure mobilization a single docking procedure for sigmoid and rectal cancer: technical notes and results. JSM Surg Oncol Res. 2016;1(1):1003.
15. Park J, You YN, Schlette E, et al. Reverse-hybrid robotic mesorectal excision for rectal cancer. Dis Colon Rectum. 2012;55(2):228–33. https://doi.org/10.1097/DCR.0b013e31823c0bd2.
16. Lim DR, Min BS, Kim MS, et al. Robotic versus laparoscopic anterior resection of sigmoid colon cancer: comparative study of long-term oncologic outcomes. Surg Endosc. 2013;27(4):1379–85. https://doi.org/10.1007/s00464-012-2619-3.
17. Panteleimonitis S, et al. Urogenital function in robotic vs laparoscopic rectal cancer surgery: a comparative study. Int J Color Dis. 2017;32:241–8.
18. Wang G, et al. Male urinary and sexual function after robotic pelvic autonomic nerve-preserving surgery for rectal cancer. Int J Med Robotics Comput Assist Surg. 2017;13:e1725.
19. Broholm M, Pommegaard H-C, Gögenür I. Possible benefits of robot-assisted rectal cancer surgery and sexual dysfunction: a systematic review and meta- analysis. Color Dis. 2014;17:375–81.
20. Van Iersel JJ, et al. Current status of laparoscopic and robotic ventral mesh rectopexy for external and internal rectal prolapse. World J Gastroenterol. 2016;22(21):4977–87.
21. D'Hoore A, et al. Long-term outcome of laparoscopic ventral rectopexy for total rectal prolapse. Br J Surg. 2004;91:1500–5. https://doi.org/10.1002/bjs.4779.
22. Vallance A, et al. A collaborative review of the current concepts and challenges of anastomotic leaks in colorectal surgery. Color Dis. 2016;19:01–012.
23. Kim JC, et al. Utility of indocyanine-green fluorescent imaging during robot-assisted sphincter-saving surgery on rectal cancer patients. Int J Med Robotics Comput Assist Surg. 2016;12:710–7.
24. Intuitive Surgical. Da Vinci vision: enhancing visualization. 2019. https://www.intuitive.com/en/products-and-services/da-vinci/vision.

Laparoscopic Colon Surgery: Education and Best Practices

8

Theodore G. Troupis, Adamantios Michalinos,
George P. Skandalakis, Phillip L. Davidson, Petros Mirilas,
and Panayiotis N. Skandalakis

8.1 Introduction

In 1991, Jacobs, Verdeja, and Goldstein were the first to perform laparoscopic colectomy [1]. Laparoscopy has been accepted by surgeons as an important treatment option that is safer than open surgery, typically has less postoperative pain, and results in less bleeding and shorter hospital stays [2]. Despite its advantages, adoption of laparoscopic colon surgery (LCS) has been relatively slow in comparison to basic laparoscopic procedures. This may be due to the long learning curve [3]. Compared with basic laparoscopic procedures, LCS presents unique technical challenges [4]. There can be difficulties with laparoscopic surgery such as a two-dimensional view, loss of hand–eye target axis, loss of tactical feedback, long inflexible instruments, less range of motion because of fixed entry points at the

T. G. Troupis (✉) · G. P. Skandalakis
Department of Anatomy, Faculty of Medicine, National and Kapodistrian University of Athens, Athens, Greece

A. Michalinos
Department of Anatomy, Faculty of Medicine, European University of Cyprus, Nicosia, Cyprus

P. L. Davidson
Doctoral Program Faculty for Business Management in Organizational Leadership and IST, University of Phoenix, College of Doctoral Studies, Phoenix, AZ, USA

P. Mirilas
'Aghia Sophia' Children's Hospital, Athens, Greece

University Paris XIII- Léonard de Vinci, Courbevoie, France

Surgical Anatomy & Technique, Emory University, Atlanta, GA, USA

P. N. Skandalakis
Anatomy and Surgical Anatomy, National and Kapodistrian University of Athens, Athens, Greece

abdomen, less degrees of freedom of laparoscopic, and camera instability [5]. The objective, therefore, is to approach the topic of education and best practices for this important surgical procedure.

8.2   Training

The training is a critical element, yet many scholars and experts have identified deficits in contemporary training, educational programs, and modules on advanced laparoscopic surgery, including LCS. According to Charron et al. [6], training in basic laparoscopy is sufficient during general surgery residency but not for advanced laparoscopy. According to their study, a resident might finish his or her residency with fewer than 30 advanced laparoscopic procedures and no more than five LCS cases. According to Gardner et al. [7], only 29% of graduating residents feel ready to perform advanced laparoscopy. In the same survey, 97% felt adequate to perform basic laparoscopy procedures. To improve their skills and fill the gap of basic training, surgeons in the United States [6] and United Kingdom [8] often pursue a laparoscopic fellowship post-residency. It may be that only through a fellowship can surgeons perform an sufficient number of cases to get trained adequately and feel "very comfortable" in LCS [9].

The learning curve for LCS has not been clearly defined, partly due to various methodologies and diverse educational populations employed in different studies. The learning curve might differ with respect to trainees' previous experience. Most authors study populations of experienced surgeons, either residents or experts. While a threshold of 50 laparoscopic colon resections is often set arbitrarily, other studies report between 10 and 70 operations should be enough to acquire the required skills for LCS. According to Luglio et al. [10], the learning curve is defined by a personal feeling of confidence and independence and a trend to limit postoperative complications, conversion rate, and operative time.

Tekkis et al. [11], using multidimensional statistical analysis of operative time, conversion rates, complications postoperatively, and rates of readmission, suggested that the learning curve required 55 procedures for right-sided colectomies and 62 for left-sided colectomies. However, that number cannot be considered an absolute, as multiple factor, such as clinical and task efficiency as well as patient outcomes can vary considerably. In a more recent study, Barrie et al. [12] specifically looked at studies that offered a specific number of procedures as the determinant for appraising the learning curve. The findings suggested the learning curve involves many variables. Even the description is poorly defined as were definitions of supervision and mentoring. Factors used to measure proficiency varied, so the attempt to use a single factor to quantify the learning curve is considered to be simplistic.

The discussion of a metric that could be used as a way of measuring proficiency is relevant to a discussion of the best practices in the teaching and education of surgeons related to LCS. However, metrics from traditional studies may be difficult to apply to LCS. As noted previously, the classical method of surgical technique mentoring ("See one, do one, teach one") may not be the best practice for the complexities involved in LCS. One example of differences is psychomotor skills.

Psychomotor skills necessary for LCS are different than those for open surgery; however, those skills follow the same educational principles as described by Fitts and Posner's three-stage motor skill acquisition model [13]. According to this model, in the first stage (cognitive stage), the learner intellectualizes the task and can perform those tasks only through a strictly conscious process. Subsequently, the procedure is carried out in distinct, separated, and nonrhythmic steps. Later, the learner reaches the second stage (integrative stage), in which knowledge is used as a more appropriate motor behavior. The learner still acts consciously, but is able to execute continuously and in fewer steps. In the third stage (autonomous stage), practice gradually results in smooth and rhythmic performance and the learner can perform unconsciously, thus he is liberated to concentrate on other aspects of the operation. Thousands of repetitions of the same task are required; still, this might be impossible inside an operating theatre [14]. This is a good description of how working memory moves from explicit to implicit memory.

The challenge is that several different memory systems are involved. While training surgeons involve time-tested methods, the "normal" memory systems involved may be different, or balanced differently. For example, in things performed every day, individuals might have a list of items in semantic memory, items such as computer passwords on PIN numbers. These are recalled on an "as-needed" basis [15]. When ideas are described to another person, the ability to recall and verbally describe the information is part of our explicit or "declarative" memory [16]. The memory system that controls the data flow in and out is working memory [15], and working memory pulls information from learned or semantic memory when needed. However, when learning something that requires physical performance, motor memory becomes involved. This is defined as implicit or procedural memory. It is enhanced through repetition as a skilled dancer will repeat the same moves repeatedly until perfected. The problem arises with LCS in that what is being learned through repetition can conflict with procedural memories learned from nonlaparoscopic surgical procedures. The dissonance between what has been learned in a traditional manner and what is being learned in LCS training requires a longer period of learning.

New technologies combined with older educational modalities might be the answer. Practice in "surgical boxes," animal models, and cadavers are old and established modalities, also applicable to LCS education. Virtual simulators are an evolution of practice boxes. Simulators also present new and unique characteristics like metrics calculation [17] that provide novel educational tools to the trainers.

8.3   Training Modalities

8.3.1   Video Training

Video training is the usual initial step in laparoscopic training, including training in LCS [7]. Through video training, trainees can appreciate, repetitively if necessary, operation steps and various surgical maneuvers. Videos are often explained by a trainer, who will add personal perspective and answer questions. They also have unique advantages including high variety and availability. Trainees can watch them outside training program hours, allowing time for other activities. A number of electronic sources provide free, high-quality surgical videos [18]. Research has involved attempts to enrich video training experience. Sugamoto et al. [19] suggested audio recording of the operation, alongside with video recording to combine surgeon's thoughts with operative actions, while Nauman et al. [20] suggested that editing of videos taken of residents enhances their active role in the operation and increases active learning.

Video training is an important part of optical recognition during laparoscopic surgery. Visual perceptual illusion is a known major error source during laparoscopic cholecystectomy accounting for 97% of errors, and this might be also true during LCS [21]. Optical recognition is maintained through constant practice and is almost never perfect, even among experts [22]. Video training is a part of both basic and advanced module of LCS training guidelines as developed by Society of American Gastrointestinal and Endoscopic Surgeons and American Society of Colon and Rectal Surgeons [23]. Concerns over quality of available videos have sometimes emerged. Trainers should provide themselves or suggest certain videos to trainees. Quality criteria proposed for educational videos are (1) authorship demonstration, (2) attribution, (3) disclosure, (4) comments, (5) readability, and (6) links to other videos [18]. Based on this information, basic video training should maintain its position early at education and as introduction to a more complete educational curriculum [22, 24].

8.3.2 Simulators

Box trainers are well-established simulation tools for teaching surgical residents and practicing surgeons, yet they might be inappropriate for LCS training. They are valuable for acquiring basic surgical skills during early years of residency, but not for the whole surgical operation practicing. Most surgeons interested in LCS are already experienced and have significant laparoscopic surgery skills. Therefore, box trainers do not add to their improvement. Their main advantages are low cost, ease of use, and durability [4]. Sometimes, according to the last Cochrane Database Systematic Review, box trainers might present better tactile feedback than virtual reality simulators, but technical evolution has changed that [25].

Virtual simulators are fundamental LCS educational tools. Their main advantages are high fidelity, metrics calculation, repetition, and data capture for feedback. Their main disadvantages are a less realistic tactile feedback compared to human tissue and high cost [4]. Early reports showed that training in virtual reality improved performance only in the simulator environment but not in the operating theatre [26]. A possible explanation is that trainees followed the learning curve of the simulator itself rather than the procedures. In addition, early data suffered from significant methodological defects, as experience on virtual reality simulators was still poor. Technology evolution has improved simulators' fidelity [4, 27], allowing a more realistic representation. Contemporary research work supports that skills acquired with laparoscopic simulation training are transferable to the operation theatre and that practice on simulator improves surgical skills and patients' care [14, 23, 28–31].

Simulation is beneficial for all training levels. As younger trainees are more familiar with virtual reality through video games, simulation might be beneficial even for novices [27, 32]. Salkini and Hamilton [33] stated that the younger the trainee, the faster the acquisition of surgical skills; therefore, laparoscopic education, at least basic skills training, should start early during residency. Simulators can calculate metrics useful both for training and evaluation. Basic calculated metrics are operative time, instrument path length, and smoothness of the trajectory of the instrument. Neary et al. [29] evaluated residents and experts practicing on simulators and demonstrated that those metrics are strongly correlated with the experience of the trainee. Metrics can therefore be used for evaluation. The same conclusions have been reached by other researchers [4, 30, 34]. Surgical results from a simulated operation can be helpful in trainee evaluation. Information such as specimen length, surgical margins, retrieved lymph nodes, geometry of the anastomosis, and surgical errors such as bowel injury, ureters injury, or practicing improper tension can all be collected in the simulated environment [30]. Neary et al. [29] also proved that apart from simulator calculated metrics, the number of surgical errors is also correlated with trainee's operative experience. Those results should be interpreted with caution as most simulators can generate only one environment and cannot represent human variability. Simulators also have an inherently longer learning curve and improvement reflects trainee's familiarization with the simulator.

Trainee's progress corresponds to shorter operative time, less surgical errors, and a more successful completion of task. Virtual simulation training improves the total operative time and the instruments' path length significantly, but improvement is less significant when it comes to surgical errors and achievement of quality measures, such as margins and adequacy of anastomosis [30, 35]. In seeking to determine which metrics demonstrated construct validity for virtual reality training in LCS, there were eight procedure-specific metrics noted out of 14 studied. Those attributes with the greatest statistical significance ($p < 0.01$) included dissection of the inferior mesenteric artery, accuracy of the peritoneal/medial mobilization, and reduced instrument path length.

Several other markers of better patient care seem improved after simulation training such as less need for expert assistance, shorter postoperative stay, less intraoperative bleeding, and less need for blood transfusion [36]. This seems rational as psychomotor skills improvement would reflect more on total operative time or path length. According to a recent meta–analysis, training simulators improve knowledge of the surgical operation, surgical skills, operative time, process, outcome, behavior time, behavior process, and patients' treatment and care [32]. In addition, because simulators capture data and produce metrics, they are useful for self-evaluation and trainees can review their performance later. Finally, they are useful for evaluation of trainees with different educational modalities, such as cadavers [37, 38].

The main disadvantages of training on simulators are high cost and a long learning curve. While laparoscopic stimulators tend to have a high front-end cost, their maintenance cost is low [27] and technological evolution constantly increases their fidelity. Also, cheaper "home-made" simulators have been used. For example, Khine et al. [39] built a laparoscopic trainer box for local shops and a high-definition web camera, purchased online. The training box is both lightweight and inexpensive and offers a workable alternative for more expensive equipment. In a more recent effort in Australia, a team developed a training box that utilized a personal smartphone [40] for the camera. These innovation solutions provide inexpensive and workable solutions when the more expensive equipment is too costly or simply unavailable. The efficacy of these homegrown systems has not yet been proven [41].

Virtual reality simulators are more effective than traditional training or nonstimulation modalities such as box trainers or videos [25, 42]. In the future, training on simulators will help surgeons become better trained and is expected to decrease the cost of their training while offering better surgical results, including shorter postoperative stay and fewer complications [36]. Until such time as more systems become available are lower prices, creative approaches to low-cost simulators will continue. It is worth nothing that Zendejas et al. [43], after an extensive systematic review of the literature, reported that while there is a belief that higher fidelity simulators (also more expensive) are more effective as training tools, the majority of studies concluded that simulators with lower fidelity (and lower costs) were similarly effective.

8.3.3   Animal Models and Cadavers

8.3.3.1 Animals

LCS training takes place also with cadaveric and animal models. Advantages are cadavers' high fidelity, realistic representation of anatomy, and ability of trainees to perform whole operations rather than isolated parts. Their main disadvantages are nonrealistic tissue sensation as compared to human tissue, nonhuman-like color, lack of bleeding, bad odor, high cost, major concerns for disease transmission, and difficulties with preservation [44]. Although animals' anatomy is different than humans', training on animal models offers better tissue sensation, the capability to practice and manage hemostasis that other training models like video training and simulation training cannot offer [14, 45–49]. The most commonly used animal models are the canine and porcine model. The canine colon presents highest similarity to human colon. The porcine model, instead, is appropriate for left colectomy and low anterior resections [50, 51].

Significant ethical issues exist concerning the use of animals for training in surgery as they usually lead to animals' death and significant pain. Legal and ethical issues raise a major concern in the medical community concerning the use of animals for training purposes [52, 53]. The moral principles of Russel and Burch [54], Dawkins [55], and Bishop and Nolen [56] highlight the challenges of the use of animals for educational and training purposes. To overcome animal training issues and concerns, trainees propose several alternative solutions. For example, Waseda et al. [57] proposed a training model consisting of an artificial, human-like abdominal wall and animal organs. According to their study, this model is highly realistic, facilitating many abdominal operations. It is also cheaper than animal models because the abdominal wall is reusable.

8.3.3.2 Cadavers

Unlike training on animals, different operations can be practiced on a single cadaver [58]. In most studies, participants believe that both cadaveric and animal models are realistic, have the same training value, and offer adequate training for surgical skills acquisition [48, 49]. The basic training curriculum of the American Society of Colon and Rectal Surgeons and the curriculum of the Society of American Gastrointestinal and Endoscopic Surgeons for LCS include practicing on a porcine model, while the advanced curricula of both societies include practicing on a cadaveric model [23]. Notably cadavers have been used in LCS for education and research very early after its introduction [59]. Use of cadavers is an attractive option and an important factor for choosing a training course [60]. According to Levine et al., cadavers have educational value in both basic and advanced surgical skills acquisition [37].

Comparison between simulators and cadavers or animal models is difficult. LeBlanc et al. [47] performed studies comparing training in cadavers and animal models for LCS. In their studies, they compared educational value, trainees' satisfaction, surgical errors, and various surgical skills. According to LeBlanc et al. [47], training on a cadaveric model is more difficult, yet it offers more satisfaction to the trainee. Surgical errors are similar for both models.

Sharma and Horgan [61] conducted a study comparing performance of trainees of various levels (experts, residents, and medical students) in surgical tasks performed on cadaveric model and high-fidelity laparoscopic simulators. In their study, all categories scored better on cadaveric models in many tasks, including proper instruments use, tissue handling, tactile feedback, replication of operative steps, understanding of anatomy, dissection of tissue plane, harmonic teamwork, and leadership. It was only experts whose performance was the same across both models.

There is a cost difference as well between animal, cadaver, and simulator training. In a study by Van Bruwaene et al. [62], a comparison was made between a control group (who had no additional training), a group using cadaver organs for training, and a virtual reality training. The individuals were evaluated against a baseline, and the results indicated that the group trained on the cadaver organs worked significantly faster (posttest) than the simulation group, and the simulation group never outperformed the control group. At the same time, the use of cadavers or porcine models is significantly less expensive. Samia et al. [63] also noted the typically lower costs and lower maintenance. However, both Van Bruwaene et al. [62] and Samia et al. [63] discussed the overall high costs of surgical training and the difficulty of separating different cost aspects of that training.

8.4 Tutorials

Considering limited presence of LCS in clinical practice and the heterogeneity of the training population, it is difficult to establish a single tutorial for LCS. Educational needs vary across different levels of trainees and also across different educational systems and countries. Scholars need to design different tutorials for residents, fellows, novice surgeons, or expert surgeons. Experience is still limited and long-term training results are awaited. A realistic tutorial should not be a "one size fits all" but it should consider number of participants, their level of education, their pre-educational experience, and their professional status. LCS training should also be adapted to financial and organizing capabilities of the organizer and institution to maintain its effectiveness and viability [36]. Different educational modalities should be combined to constitute an adequate tutorial. The "golden rule" between different modalities remains under investigation. Different institutions follow different rules, often defined empirically or by non-evidenced studies. Concerning residents, Gardner et al. [7] performed a survey at faculty members and surgery trainees attempting to define the ideal curriculum. Interestingly, answers of both groups were similar (Table 8.1). A combination of educational modalities is necessary for residents' training starting from video training and finishing with supervised operation.

A different tutorial should be designed for fellows because they already have operative experience and possess basic laparoscopic surgical skills. For this educational group, out-of-operative room modalities lose their significance and in-room experience is of primary importance. A combined curriculum including simulation and supervised operation seems an appropriate educational method [9]. Most residents prefer to follow a fellowship to improve their skills in LCS [6–8]. According to some authors, operational exposure under supervision and mentoring is equally good with structured learning, without the need for sophisticated educational modalities [10]. Distribution of educational resources between residents and fellows is a concern. Although many would believe that such a coexistence would be to residents' encumbrance, literature data are scarce to support or reject this point of view [6, 64, 65].

Table 8.1 Gardner et al. [7] survey on definition of curriculum for laparoscopic colon surgery training

	Residents (%)	Faculty members (%)
Clinical environment	56%	48
Live animal models	11	12
Cadaver laboratory	8	6
Virtual reality simulator	7	8
Physical model simulator	6	11
Videos	6	9
Didactic lectures	6	6

Experienced surgeons but nonexperts in LCS constitute a special population of trainees. Although they have significant experience in both laparoscopic and open surgery, they are of a more advanced age and thus follow different educational and learning mechanisms. Furthermore, they usually practice in a hospital and they cannot be absent for a long time. Therefore, a fellowship would not be a preferred option to develop their surgical skills and knowledge in LCS. For this educational population, existence of a mentor trained in LCS seems essential. To promote a wider adoption of LCS, England established the National Training program. This program followed a preclinical phase alongside with a clinical phase that consisted of independent supervised operations. For the clinical phase of the program, trainer–trainee pairs were created. Upon completion of each case, global assessment forms were submitted by trainees and trainers that evaluated the progress of the trainee and the educational value of the program. Those forms were used for feedback and also for fund distribution, as they evaluated quantity and quality of education [66]. A tele-mentoring program structured in three phases has also been described by Schlachta et al. in Canada [67]. During the first phase of the program, the mentor must be physically present and scrubbed. In the second phase, the mentor must be physically present but not scrubbed, and in the third phase, he or she would only tele-mentor the operation through a network connecting the two hospitals that participated in the training program. Authors dispute the utility of tele-mentoring programs for large, under populated areas. Finally, Dominguez et al. [68] reported that the integration of a surgeon who is trained in minimally invasive techniques in an established practice team can increase the quality of laparoscopically performed operations and improve the outcome of the operations. In a 4-year period, laparoscopically performed operations increased by 300% with LCS cases increasing from 25.6% to 52.3% because of adding an expert in the team. The new colleague acted like a mentor for other surgeons. Data analysis showed that mentoring from a trained colleague acted stronger than other educational modalities like training videos or short training sessions.

8.5 Operating Room Experience: The Role of Hand-Assisted Laparoscopic Colectomy

Despite wide acceptance of advanced laparoscopic surgery, trainees' operative experience in LCS remains suboptimal [3, 4]. This is a multifactorial phenomenon. Increased complexity of the operation, diminished trainer's availability, operative time, and safety concerns result in limited residents' operative experience. LCS is not sufficiently taught during surgery training or is mainly offered to fellows rather than residents. Charron et al. [6] reported that residents on average perform only four laparoscopic colectomies during their residency, while colorectal fellows perform almost 50. The laparoscopic experience a new surgeon gains during residency is limited for advanced laparoscopic surgery, including LCS [64]. However, introducing LCS early during residency is more efficient in decreasing complications, conversions, and readmission rates [69].

Miller et al. [70] published data on training on single incision laparoscopic surgery (SILS) colectomy in a selected population. With this technique, surgeons must take more operative steps, which makes it more difficult than two or three port LCS but no additional morbidity, mortality, conversion rates, or hospital stay were encountered. Hand-assisted laparoscopic colectomy (HALC) is often considered an introduction to straight laparoscopic colectomy [60]. Data show that at the end of their learning curve, surgeons choose only one of the two procedures for their practice [71]. LeBlanc et al. [72] compared the two procedures during a simulator course and found that their metrics are quite different. Authors found that HALC is a shorter procedure in terms of total time and hand motion. Most time was gained during mobilization of splenic flexure and sigmoid colon. Surgical errors performed were similar. Champagne et al. [71] have doubted educational value of HALC as an introduction to straight laparoscopic colectomy as they believe they are different procedures with different surgical techniques and probably different indications and contradictions. Some authors [71, 73] question the educational value of short curricula versus complete educational LCS programs during residency or fellowship. Longer structured education programs are superior overshorter courses. Many surgeons, who did not receive adequate training in LCS during residency or fellowship, choose to receive training later during their practice. These later training programs do not offer the same value as a 1 or 2 years' structured educational and training program. Surgeons who train at a later stage of their career are usually older with significant experience in laparoscopic and open colon surgery and thus a different population than residents or fellows who have different training and learning needs. Nevertheless, even short educational courses are better than noting and can add value to surgeons who would like to perform LCS instead of open surgery [60].

8.6   Conclusion: A Complete Curriculum

LCS training is a complex process. Experience in basic laparoscopic surgery is a prerequisite for a surgeon to be able to perform LCS, which is a more complex and demanding surgical procedure. A variety of educational modalities are available for LCS training like video training, box trainer, simulators, cadavers, and animal models. Those are complementary as no single educational modality can substitute the others and support by itself a complete educational curriculum and training program. Accomplishment of certain educational targets is not a goal per se but rather acts as a prologue to complex in operation training. Thus, a complete preoperational curriculum should include basic training with simple modalities such as box training or physical simulators, advanced training with high-fidelity simulators, and finally practicing of the whole surgical procedure using cadaveric or animal models [4, 14, 23, 27]. Adaptability is essential as different educational groups have different needs and different teaching institutions afford different educational resources and follow a different educational philosophy and protocol. Regardless of training modality or training population, a complete curriculum to be effective should follow certain educational and psychological principles to enhance trainees' motivation, offer adequate training time, and provide the necessary human and material resources. Furthermore, feedback, clear performance targets, repetitive practice, continuous education, and recertification processes are necessary to ensure quality of care and promote for continuous improvement and learning [74].

Healthcare needs and priorities of healthcare practitioners, availability of resources, and patients' demands and increased awareness have a significant impact on training modalities and educational curricula. A structured training program should be attractive to healthcare stakeholders and not only counter the needs of the surgical community. Contemporary surgeons and surgical communities need to identify those training and educational models that meet societal needs and healthcare targets other than merely their and leaders by proving its superiority and durability not only in scientific or educational terms but also in terms of organizing and financial benefits [36].

Multimodality, structured training is superior to basic surgical training. It shortens educational time in operation theatre, decreases complications, and ultimately costs [14, 75]. Details of an educational program should be adapted to trainees' population, educational, financial, organizational priorities, and resources. The ideal educational and training curriculum should be a balance among academia and educational needs, technology evolvement, administrative resources, healthcare institutional goals, and patients' wellness.

References

1. Jacobs M, Verdeja JC, Goldstein HS. Minimally invasive colon resection (laparoscopic colectomy). Surg Laparosc Endosc. 1991;1(3):144–50.
2. Bardakcioglu O, Khan A, Aldridge C, Chen J. Growth of laparoscopic colectomy in the United States: analysis of regional and socioeconomic factors over time. Ann Surg. 2013;258(2):270–4.
3. Schlachta CM, Mamazza J, Seshadri PA, Cadeddu M, Gregoire R, Poulin EC. Defining a learning curve for laparoscopic colorectal resections. Dis Colon Rectum. 2001;44(2):217–22.
4. Celentano V. Need for simulation in laparoscopic colorectal surgery training. World J Gastrointest Surg. 2015;7(9):185–9.
5. Heemskerk J, Zandbergen R, Maessen JG, Greve JWM, Bouvy ND. Advantages of advanced laparoscopic systems. Surg Endosc. 2006;20(5):730–3.
6. Charron P, Campbell R, Dejesus S, Gallagher J, Williamson P, Ferrara A. The gap in laparoscopic colorectal experience between colon and rectal and general surgery residency training programs. Dis Colon Rectum. 2007;50(12):2023–31. discussion 2031
7. Gardner AK, Willis RE, Dunkin BJ, Van Sickle K, Brown K, Truitt M, Uecker J, Gentry L, Scott D. What do residents need to be competent laparoscopic and endoscopic surgeons? Surg Endosc. 2015;30(7):3050–9.
8. Williams GL, Sagar PM, McAllister I, Gonsalves S. The laparoscopic colorectal fellowships are popular, educational and produce competent laparoscopic surgeons. Color Dis. 2009;11(5):519–21.
9. Stein S, Stulberg J, Champagne B. Learning laparoscopic colectomy during colorectal residency: what does it take and how are we doing? Surg Endosc. 2012;26(2):488–92.
10. Luglio G, De Palma GD, Tarquini R, Giglio M, Sollazo V, Esposito E, Spadarella E, Peltrini R, Liccardo F, Bucci L. Laparoscopic colorectal surgery in learning curve: Role of implementation of a standardized technique and recovery protocol. A cohort study. Ann Med Surg (Lond). 2015;4(2):89–94.

11. Tekkis PP, Senagore AJ, Delaney CP, Fazio VW. Evaluation of the learning curve in laparoscopic colorectal surgery: comparison of right-sided and left- sided resections. Ann Surg. 2005;242(1):83–91.

12. Barrie J, Jayne DG, Wright J, Murray CJC, Collinson FJ, Pavitt SH. Attaining surgical competency and its implications in surgical clinical trial design: a systematic review of the learning curve in laparoscopic and robot-assisted laparoscopic colorectal cancer surgery. Ann Surg Oncol. 2014;21(3):829–40.

13. Fitts P, Posner M. Human performance. Brooks/Cole: Belmont; 1967.

14. Reznick RK, MacRae H. Teaching surgical skills--changes in the wind. N Engl J Med. 2006;355(25):2664–9.

15. Gade M, Druey MD, Souze AS, Oberauer K. Interference within the between declarative and procedural representations in working memory. J Mem Lang. 2014;76(October):174–94.

16. Masters RSW, Poolton JM, Abernethy B, Patil NG. Implicit learning of movement skills for surgery. ANZ J Surg. 2008;78(12):1062–4.

17. Oostema JA, Abdel MP, Gould JC. Time-efficient laparoscopic skills assessment using an augmented- reality simulator. Surg Endosc. 2008;22(12):2621–4.

18. Dinscore A, Andres A. Surgical videos online: a survey of prominent sources and future trends. Med Ref Serv Q. 2010;29(1):10–27.

19. Sugamoto Y, Hamamoto Y, Kimura M, Fukunga T, Tasaki K, Asai Y, Takeshita N, Maruyama T, Hosokawa T, Tamachi T, Aouyama H, Matsubara H. A novel method for real-time audio recording with intraoperative video. J Surg Educ. 2015;72(5):795–802.

20. Naumann DN, Bowley DM, McArthur DR. The director's cut - video editing as a training modality for minimally invasive surgery. Minim Invasive Ther Allied Technol. 2014;23(3):188–9.

21. Way LW, Stewart L, Gantert W, Liu K, Lee C, Whang K, Hunter J. Causes and prevention of laparoscopic bile duct injuries: analysis of 252 cases from a human factors and cognitive psychology perspective. Ann Surg. 2003;237(4):460–9.

22. Tolerton SK, Hugh TJ, Cosman PH. The production of audiovisual teaching tools in minimally invasive surgery. J Surg Educ. 2012;69(3):404–6.

23. Fleshman J, Marcello P, Stamos MJ, Wexner SD. American Society of Colon and Rectal Surgeons (ASCRS), Society of American Gastrointestinal and Endoscopic Surgeons (SAGES). Focus group on laparoscopic colectomy education as endorsed by the American Society of Colon and Rectal Surgeons (ASCRS) and the Society of American Gastrointestinal and Endoscopic Surgeons (SAGES). Dis Colon Rectum. 2006;49(7):945–9.

24. Abdelsattar JM, Pandian TK, Finnesgard EJ, El Khatib M, Rowse P, Buckarama E, Gas B, Heller S, Farley D. Do you see what I see? How we use video as an adjunct to general surgery resident education. J Surg Educ. 2015;72(6):e145–50.

25. Nagendran M, Gurusamy KS, Aggarwal R, Loizidou M, Davidson BR. Virtual reality training for surgical trainees in laparoscopic surgery. Cochrane Database Syst Rev. 2013;8:CD006575.

26. Ahlberg G, Heikkinen T, Iselius L, Leijonmarck C-E, Rutqvist J, Arvidsson D. Does training in a virtual reality simulator improve surgical performance? Surg Endosc. 2002;16(1):126–9.

27. Bashankaev B, Baido S, Wexner SD. Review of available methods of simulation training to facilitate surgical education. Surg Endosc. 2011;25(1):28–35.

28. Seymour NE, Gallagher AG, Roman SA, O'Brien M, Bansal P, Andersen D, Satava R. Virtual reality training improves operating room performance: results of a randomized, double-blinded study. Ann Surg. 2002;236(4):458. -463-464

29. Neary PC, Boyle E, Delaney CP, Senagore AJ, Keane FBV, Gallagher AG. Construct validation of a novel hybrid virtual-reality simulator for training and assessing laparoscopic colectomy; results from the first course for experienced senior laparoscopic surgeons. Surg Endosc. 2008;22(10):2301–9.

30. Essani R, Scriven RJ, McLarty AJ, Merriam LT, Ahn H, Bergamaschi R. Simulated laparoscopic sigmoidectomy training: responsiveness of surgery residents. Dis Colon Rectum. 2009;52(12):1956–61.

31. Stelzer MK, Abdel MP, Sloan MP, Gould JC. Dry lab practice leads to improved laparoscopic performance in the operating room. J Surg Res. 2009;154(1):163–6.
32. Zendejas B, Brydges R, Hamstra SJ, Cook DA. State of the evidence on simulation-based training for laparoscopic surgery: a systematic review. Ann Surg. 2013;257(4):586–93.
33. Salkini MW, Hamilton AJ. The effect of age on acquiring laparoscopic skills. J Endourol. 2010;24(3):377–9.
34. LeBlanc F, Champagne BJ, Augestad KM, Neary P, Senagore A, Ellis C, Delaney C. A comparison of human cadaver and augmented reality simulator models for straight laparoscopic colorectal skills acquisition training. J Am Coll Surg. 2010;211(2):250–5.
35. Lee M, Savage J, Dias M, Berggren P, Winter M. Box, cable and smartphone: a simple laparoscopic trainer. Clin Teach. 2015;12(6):384–8.
36. Matsiota E. Laparoscopic colectomy training: a quasi experimental comparison of simulators to traditional training. 2015. http://media.proquest.com/media/pq/classic/doc/3787326151/fmt/ai/rep/NPDF?_s=jP0cUUpvVOKeJT1MmA QFuqQQRww%3D.
37. Levine RL, Kives S, Cathey G, Blinchevsky A, Acland R, Thomson R, Pasic R. The use of lightly embalmed (fresh tissue) cadavers for resident laparoscopic training. J Minim Invasive Gynecol. 2006;13(5):451–6.
38. Khine M, Leung E, Morran C, Muthukumarasamy G. Homemade laparoscopic simulators for surgical trainees. Clin Teach. 2011;8(2):118–21.
39. Gilbody J, Prasthofer AW, Ho K, Costa ML. The use and effectiveness of cadaveric workshops in higher surgical training: a systematic review. Ann R Coll Surg Engl. 2011;93(5):347–52.
40. Zendejas B, Wang AT, Brydges R, Hamstra SJ, Cook DA. Costs: the missing outcome in simulation-based medical education research: a systematic review. Surgery. 2013;153(2):160–76.
41. Aslam A, Nason GJ, Giri SK. Homemade laparoscopic surgical simulator: a cost-effective solution to the challenge of acquiring laparoscopic skills? Ir J Med Sci. 2016;185(4):791–6.
42. Larsen CR, Soerensen JL, Grantcharov TP, Dalsgaard R, Schouenborg L, Ottosen C, Schroeder B, Ottosen B. Effect of virtual reality training on laparoscopic surgery: randomised controlled trial. BMJ. 2009;338:b1802.
43. Van Bruwaene S, Schijven MP, Napolitano D, De Win G, Miserez M. Porcine cadaver organ or virtual-reality simulation training for laparoscopic cholecystectomy: a randomized, controlled trial. J Surg Educ. 2015;72(3):483–90.
44. Hayashi S, Naito M, Kawata S, Qu N, Hatayama N, Hirai S, Itho M. History and future of human cadaver preservation for surgical training: from formalin to saturated salt solution method. Anat Sci Int. 2015;91(1):1–7.
45. Udomsawaengsup S, Pattana-arun J, Tansatit T, Pungapong S, Navicharern P, Sirichindakul B, Nonthassot B, Park-art R, Sriassadeporn S, Kyttayakerrana K, Wongsaisuwan M, Rojanaskul A. Minimally invasive surgery training in soft cadaver (MIST-SC). J Med Assoc Thai. 2005;88(Suppl 4):S189–94.
46. Giger U, Frésard I, Häfliger A, Bergmann M, Krähenbühl L. Laparoscopic training on Thiel human cadavers: a model to teach advanced laparoscopic procedures. Surg Endosc. 2008;22(4):901–6.
47. Leblanc F, Senagore AJ, Ellis CN, Champagne B, Augestad K, Neary P, Delaney C. Hand-assisted laparoscopic sigmoid colectomy skills acquisition: augmented reality simulator versus human cadaver training models. J Surg Educ. 2010;67(4):200–4.
48. Wyles SM, Miskovic D, Ni Z, Acheson A, Maxwell C, Longman R, Cecil T, Coleman M, Horgan A, Hanna G. Analysis of laboratory-based laparoscopic colorectal surgery workshops within the English National Training Programme. Surg Endosc. 2011;25(5):1559–66.
49. Stefanidis D, Yonce TC, Green JM, Coker AP. Cadavers versus pigs: which are better for procedural training of surgery residents outside the OR? Surgery. 2013;154(1):34–7.
50. Böhm B, Milsom JW, Kitago K, Brand M, Fazio VW. Laparoscopic oncologic total abdominal colectomy with intraperitoneal stapled anastomosis in a canine model. J Laparoendosc Surg. 1994;4(1):23–30.

51. Böhm B, Milsom JW. Animal models as educational tools in laparoscopic colorectal surgery. Surg Endosc. 1994;8(6):707–13.
52. Byrne P. Teaching laparoscopic surgery. Practice on live animals is illegal. BMJ. 1994;308(6941):1435.
53. Rollin BE. The regulation of animal research and the emergence of animal ethics: a conceptual history. Theor Med Bioeth. 2006;27(4):285–304.
54. Russel W, Buch R. The principle of humane experimental technique. London: Methuen; 1959.
55. Dawkins M. Animal suffering: the science of animal welfare. Springer Science & Business Media; 2012.
56. Bishop LJ, Nolen AL. Animals in research and education: ethical issues. Kennedy Inst Ethics J. 2001;11(1):91–112.
57. Waseda M, Inaki N, Mailaender L, Buess GF. An innovative trainer for surgical procedures using animal organs. Minim Invasive Ther Allied Technol. 2005;14(4):262–6.
58. Sharma M, Macafee D, Horgan AF. Basic laparoscopic skills training using fresh frozen cadaver: a randomized controlled trial. Am J Surg. 2013;206(1):23–31.
59. Milsom JW, Böhm B, Decanini C, Fazio VW. Laparoscopic oncologic proctosigmoidectomy with low colorectal anastomosis in a cadaver model. Surg Endosc. 1994;8(9):1117–23.
60. Ross HM, Simmang CL, Fleshman JW, Marcello PW. Adoption of laparoscopic colectomy: results and implications of ASCRS hands-on course participation. Surg Innov. 2008;15(3):179–83.
61. Sharma M, Horgan A. Comparison of fresh-frozen cadaver and high-fidelity virtual reality simulator as methods of laparoscopic training. World J Surg. 2012;36(8):1732–7.
62. Shanmugan S, Leblanc F, Senagore AJ, Ellis CN, Stein SL, Khan S, et al. Virtual reality simulator training for laparoscopic colectomy: what metrics have construct validity? Dis Colon Rectum. 2014;57(2):210–2144.
63. Samia H, Khan S, Lawrence J, Delaney CP. Simulation and its role in training. Clin Colon Rectal Surg. 2013;26(1):47–55.
64. Rattner DW, Apelgren KN, Eubanks WS. The need for training opportunities in advanced laparoscopic surgery. Surg Endosc. 2001;15(10):1066–70.
65. Reynolds FD, Goudas L, Zuckerman RS, Gold MS, Heneghan S. A rural, community-based program can train surgical residents in advanced laparoscopy. J Am Coll Surg. 2003;197(4):620–3.
66. Coleman MG, Hanna GB, Kennedy R, National Training Programme Lapco. The National Training Programme for laparoscopic colorectal surgery in England: a new training paradigm. Color Dis. 2011;13(6):614–6.
67. Schlachta CM, Sorsdahl AK, Kent SA, Lefebvre KL, McCune ML, Jayaraman S. A model for longitudinal mentoring and telementoring of laparoscopic colon surgery. Surg Endosc. 2009;23(7):1634–8.
68. Dominguez EP, Barrat C, Shaffer L, Gruner R, Whisler D, Taylor P. Minimally invasive surgery adoption into an established surgical practice: impact of a fellowship- trained colleague. Surg Endosc. 2013;27(4):1267–72.
69. Daetwiler S, Guller U, Schob O, Adamina M. Early introduction of laparoscopic sigmoid colectomy during residency. Br J Surg. 2007;94(5):634–41.
70. Miller S, Causey MW, Damle A, Maykel J, Steele S. Single-incision laparoscopic colectomy: training the next generation. Surg Endosc. 2013;27(5):1784–90.
71. Champagne BJ, Lee EC, Valerian B, Armstrong D, Ambroze W, Orangio G. A novel end point to assess a resident's ability to perform hand-assisted versus straight laparoscopy for left colectomy: is there really a difference? J Am Coll Surg. 2008;207(4):554–9.
72. Leblanc F, Delaney CP, Ellis CN, Neary PC, Champagne BJ, Senagore AJ. Hand-assisted versus straight laparoscopic sigmoid colectomy on a training simulator: what is the difference? A stepwise comparison of hand-assisted versus straight laparoscopic sigmoid colectomy performance on an augmented reality simulator. World J Surg. 2010;34(12):2909–14.

73. Zimmerman H, Latifi R, Dehdashti B, Ong E, Jie T, Galvani C, Waer A, Wynne J, Biffar D, Gruessner R. Intensive laparoscopic training course for surgical residents: program description, initial results, and requirements. Surg Endosc. 2011;25(11):3636–41.
74. Stefanidis D, Heniford BT. The formula for a successful laparoscopic skills curriculum. Arch Surg. 2009;144(1):77–82; discussion 82
75. Lin E, Szomstein S, Addasi T, Galati-Burke L, Turner JW, Tiszenkel HI. Model for teaching laparoscopic colectomy to surgical residents. Am J Surg. 2003;186(1):45–8.

Anesthesia in Laparoscopic Colorectal Surgery

Amalia Douma, Alexander-Michael Nixon, and Ifigeneia Grigoriadou

9.1 Introduction

Since its introduction, four decades ago, laparoscopic surgery has established itself as an attractive alternative to traditional open abdominal procedures. This is evident in colorectal surgery where over the past 20 years laparoscopy is gradually replacing traditional procedures in a variety of benign and malignant conditions. Benefits of this minimally invasive approach include earlier mobilization, better cosmetic results, shorter hospital stays, and limited surgical trauma. As experience and familiarity with the technologies involved has increased amongst practitioners so has the scope of laparoscopic surgery. Furthermore, better understanding of the physiological changes that occur during establishment of pneumoperitoneum has rendered significant comorbidities such as coronary heart disease or chronic obstructive pulmonary disease (COPD) manageable and are not anymore considered absolute contraindications to laparoscopy.

In this chapter, we describe alterations in physiological parameters during pneumoperitoneum and patient positioning and highlight specific considerations in the anesthesiological management of colorectal surgery.

A. Douma · I. Grigoriadou
Department of Anaesthesiology, General Hospital of Athens "G. Gennimatas", Athens, Greece

A.-M. Nixon (✉)
Third Department of Surgery, General Hospital of Athens "G. Gennimatas", Athens, Greece

© The Editor(s) (if applicable) and The Author(s), under exclusive license to Springer Nature Switzerland AG 2021
G. Kouraklis, E. (J.) Matsiota (eds.), *Laparoscopic Colon Surgery*,
https://doi.org/10.1007/978-3-030-56728-6_9

9.2   Insufflation of CO$_2$

Establishment of pneumoperitoneum is the initial step in any laparoscopic procedure and results in guarantying adequate visualization of the abdominal cavity and the requisite space for handling surgical instruments and manipulating tissues. Pneumoperitoneum is provided by the insufflation of gas in the abdominal cavity, which in turn causes an increase in intra-abdominal pressure (IAP). Normal IAP has a range of 0–5 mmHg while most laparoscopic procedures require a pressure of at least 10 mmHg.

In the past, a variety of gaseous agents were tested for pneumoperitoneum including helium, nitrous oxide, and nitrogen which did not find favor amongst surgeons due to adverse effects such as combustion or systematic embolism [1]. Because of the physio-chemical properties of carbon dioxide (CO$_2$), CO$_2$ is the gas most commonly used as it is odorless and noncombustible. Furthermore, it reduces the duration of residual pneumoperitoneum and has minimal adverse effects when introduced in the extraperitoneal space. The disadvantages of CO2 include peritoneal irritation and elevation of PaCO$_2$ due to systemic absorption. CO$_2$ is usually insufflated at a rate of 4–6 l/min up to a pressure of 10–20 mmHg. Maintenance of pneumoperitoneum is achieved by a constant gas flow of 200–400 ml/min [2].

9.3   Pathophysiologic Changes

Prolonged elevations in IAP alter normal physiological parameters in organs and systems beyond the abdominal cavity. Normal function of different systems can be destabilized, leading to complications that can potentially affect patient morbidity and mortality [3].

9.3.1   Respiratory System

Normal respiratory function can be impaired due to a combination of elevated IAP and extreme Trendelenburg positioning [3]. Structural properties of the chest wall and the lungs such as compliance are reduced by 30–50% in healthy as well as in obese patients. Although the mechanism for this has not been fully elucidated, stiffening of the chest wall and of the lungs has been proposed as the likely cause. In addition to a decrease in compliance, pneumoperitoneum also decreases the end-expiratory lung volume [3].

Apart from its effects on the chest wall, increased IAP shifts the abdominal wall to a less compliant region of its pressure–volume curve. As a result, the abdominal wall and diaphragm stiffen and this may increase pleural pressure and pressure to the lungs [3].

Pneumoperitoneum causes a reduction in functional residual capacity (FRC), elevation of the diaphragm predisposes to atelectasis, and increased airway pressure causes changes in pulmonary ventilation and perfusion (V/Q mismatch). Ventilation strategies that are suggested to minimize the respiratory effects of pneumoperitoneum include the application of higher positive end-expiratory pressure (PEEP) as well as recruitment maneuvers in order to maintain alveoli patency.

In adults without severe comorbidities, limited elevation of IAP up to 10 mmHg does not significantly change physiological dead space or shunt in Trendelenburg (head down) or reverse Trendelenburg (head up) positioning (10–20°). Conversely, IAP above 10 mmHg increases respiratory dead space and widens the $PaCO_2$–$PetCO_2$ gradient. Increases in $PaCO_2$ are mainly the result of CO_2 absorption from the peritoneum as well as V/Q mismatch [3]. Systemic absorption of CO_2 increases with prolongation of pneumoperitoneum and with enhanced perfusion of the abdominal wall. Subcutaneous emphysema after inadvertent CO_2 leakage has also been implicated as an independent factor in CO_2 absorption [4]. Increase of $PaCO_2$ reaches a plateau after 15–30 min and depends on IAP. In laparoscopic colectomies, the steep Trendelenburg position can result in considerable V/Q mismatch causing hypoxemia and hypercapnia. In rare circumstances, edema of the upper airway and the need for immediate reintubation has been observed following prolonged steep Trendelenburg positioning [5].

9.3.2 Cardiovascular System

The cardiovascular system is not immune to physiological alterations during laparoscopic procedures. The reaction of the cardiovascular system to any type of laparoscopic surgery depends on the phase of surgery (induction of anesthesia, establishment of pneumoperitoneum, cessation of pneumoperitoneum, and recovery from anesthesia). The changes observed during induction and recovery from anesthesia are similar between laparoscopic and open surgery whereas unique conditions are observed during establishment of pneumoperitoneum [6]. The cardiovascular response during pneumoperitoneum is dependent on the type of surgery and patient characteristics. Preexisting cardiovascular disease, prescription medication, neuro-hormonal factors as well as intraoperative factors such as patient positioning, the level of IAP, CO_2 absorption, surgical technique, and the duration of the procedure modulate the effects of pneumoperitoneum [1].

The most commonly observed effects on the cardiovascular system during laparoscopy are reduced venous return due to increased IAP, increased systemic vascular resistance (SVR), and increased heart rate and mean arterial blood pressure because of neuro-hormonal stimulation [2, 7]. In addition, central venous pressure (CVP) and pulmonary capillary wedge pressure (PCWP) may increase during establishment of pneumoperitoneum [8].

The mechanism by which pneumoperitoneum affects SVR elevation is postulated to be the compression of the aorta and synchronous activation of the vasopressin and renin–angiotensin–aldosterone axis [9]. In addition, the increases in IAP lead to compression of the inferior vena cava which reduces venous return and cardiac preload [1].

The combined effects of these changes have an impact on cardiac output (CO). During low levels (7.5 mmHg) of IAP, CO has been shown to modestly increase [10]. However, over 15 mmHg CO decreases marking this as a threshold for pneumoperitoneum pressure. Previously published guidelines strongly support the application of low IAP (7.5 mmHg) during laparoscopy [11]. In our experience, the vast majority of laparoscopic procedures is concluded with IAP <15 mmHg without creating undue difficulties for the surgical team.

All of the aforementioned physiological changes have not been shown to have any considerable impact on healthy individuals but should be taken into account when dealing with patients with severe cardiovascular risk factors [12].

9.3.3 Renal Effects

Increased IAP due to pneumoperitoneum has been shown to have pathophysiological effects on renal function. The consequences of CO_2 insufflation on renal physiology and the mechanisms that produce them are under debate [13]. Even a modest IAP of 10 mmHg during laparoscopic surgery has been shown to produce transient oliguria and reduced glomerular filtration rate (GFR) and renal blood flow (RBF) [14, 15]. One proposed mechanism for these observed effects is that the combination of reduced afferent flow due to low CO and reduced efferent flow due to venous stasis results in a decreased renal perfusion gradient [16]. Experimental data on animals strongly suggest that the adverse renal effects observed are influenced by the level of intra-abdominal pressure (IAP), volume status, extent of hypercapnia, positioning, and preexisting hemodynamic and renal condition [17].

Additional factors that may affect renal function include direct compression of the renal parenchyma and renal vein, increased resistance in the renal vasculature, and release of vasoconstrictors, such as vasopressin, angiotensin II, catecholamines, and endothelin (ET)-1 [18, 19]. ET-1 is a very potent natural mammalian vasoconstrictor agent, mainly targeting the cardiovascular system and other target organs by binding to two specific receptors, ETA and ETB. The kidney is both a target organ and a major source of ET-1 production. Using an animal model, Abassi et al. suggested that a lot of the deviation from normal function observed during pneumoperitoneum may be mediated through the reduced modulated actions of ET-1 [18]. In addition, the endogenous NO system may also play a complimentary role in kidney function seen in pneumoperitoneum. Experimental data also suggests that renal reperfusion after desufflation leads to the creation of free oxygen radicals that promote renal injury [20].

The clinical significance of these findings has not been yet established. The majority of the aforementioned studies were based on animal models and it is not clear if these results can be extrapolated to patients. For example, Schafer and Krahenbuhl concluded that although good data exist to show that RBF decreases during pneumoperitoneum, this is probably inconsequential unless there is a predisposing risk factor affecting renal function [21]. After desufflation, renal function and urine output return to normal, and recent reports indicate that laparoscopy might actually be associated with a lower incidence of acute kidney injury in patients [22].

9.3.4 Cerebral Effects

Increased IAP, steep Trendelenburg position, and hypercapnia, all have independent effects on the hemodynamics of cerebral circulation. An elevated IAP causes a proportional increase in intracerebral pressure (ICP) by limiting cerebral venous drainage as a consequence of raised intrathoracic pressure [23]. Increases in IAP also interfere with cerebrospinal fluid (CSF) absorption due to elevated pressure in the lumbar venous plexus which results in inadequate venous drainage [1]. Patients vulnerable to alterations in cerebral homeostasis are those with impaired cerebral autoregulation due to head trauma.

The cerebral perfusion pressure (CPP), the driving pressure for brain perfusion, is calculated as the difference between the mean arterial pressure (MAP) and ICP. In healthy individuals, the simple equation CPP = MAP−ICP is employed to provide an approximation of CPP [24]. The exaggerated head-down position which is frequently employed in laparoscopic colorectal and prostate surgery results in increases in CVP which in turn lead to increases in ICP [25]. There is an even greater increase in the cerebral arterial pressure which counteracts the elevated levels of ICP. Theoretically, this hemodynamic deregulation can predispose to cerebral edema with negative sequelae. However, in patients without a history of head trauma, prolonged steep Trendelenburg position during laparoscopic surgery does not seem to have any significant neurological adverse effects [26].

The effects of transient increases in $PaCO_2$ during laparoscopy have been shown to have minimal effects on cerebral perfusion compared to increases in IAP and patient positioning during the procedure [27].

9.3.5 Splanchnic Effects

Elevated IAP due to pneumoperitoneum causes a decrease in hepatic blood flow. Local hypercapnia, on the other hand, results in splanchnic vasodilation. These two effects counteract one another and therefore the net effect on splanchnic circulation is minimal [28].

9.4 Positioning

In laparoscopic colectomy, the patient needs to be positioned as to allow for the passive retraction of the small intestine in an attempt to facilitate exposure of the large bowel. In the case of laparoscopic rectal surgery, the patient is placed in a steep head-down (steep Trendelenburg) position which without appropriate precautions can leave the patient at risk of inadvertently sliding off the operating table. As is the case with any open or laparoscopic procedure, appropriate padding is placed in order to avoid nerve injury.

In our experience, cross-body taping is an adequate measure to avoid mishaps during steep Trendelenburg. As a precaution, after induction of anesthesia and endotracheal intubation and before draping, the patient is positioned in the steep Trendelenburg position to evaluate any passive movement and sliding.

Most of the effects on physiology by steep Trendelenburg were reviewed in the previous paragraphs, such as the effects on CVP and ICP. However, sudden changes in patient positioning such as from steep Trendelenburg to supine can lead to abrupt hemodynamic changes such as an increase in venous return [1]. Conversely, the opposite is noted during the repositioning of the patient from supine to Trendelenburg where venous pooling occurs and there is a notable decrease in preload. For example, it has been documented that insufflation in the Trendelenburg position is accompanied by an up to 50% decline in cardiac index (CI) up to 50%, whereas no changes were observed in CI or ejection fraction with insufflation in the supine position [1]. Despite these observations, the physiological impact of positioning in laparoscopic colectomy seems to have minimal clinical significance in patients without severe comorbidities.

9.5   Immune and Stress Response

Trauma due to any cause initiates several inflammatory and inhibitory neural responses and laparoscopy-induced trauma is no exception [29, 30]. It has been suggested that surgical stress-induced responses can have a major effect on clinical outcome [31]. A salient benefit of laparoscopic surgery is a lower degree of surgical trauma due to small incisions in the abdominal wall and limited tissue manipulation. Therefore, with a reduction of surgical trauma during laparoscopy, there should be a marked decrease in the observed inflammatory response. The clinical significance of a reduced inflammatory reaction would be a lower incidence of postoperative infectious complications, as well as diminished local tumor recurrence or metastases. Several circulating inflammatory markers such as C-reactive protein and IL-6 are significantly lower with the laparoscopic approach, indicating a milder immune response [32, 33].

However, abdominal distention and the presence of CO_2 which occur during pneumoperitoneum can have an independent effect on the immune system. The peritoneal response after laparoscopic surgery seems to be characterized by a brief period of immune suppression, attributable to CO_2 insufflation. Function of inflammatory cells in the peritoneum, such as macrophages, is affected, leading to lower cytokines production and diminished phagocytosis [34]. This transient immunosuppression is not as exaggerated as in traditional laparotomy and therefore laparoscopy seems to confer a net advantage in maintaining immunological integrity [35].

9.6   Anesthetic Management

As was previously described in detail, the presence of pneumoperitoneum creates unique physiological alterations when compared to traditional open surgery and anesthesiological management needs to be tailored accordingly. Communication and coordination with the surgical team are of paramount importance especially regarding patient positioning and pneumoperitoneum settings. Comorbidities such as cardiovascular disease and COPD are not considered absolute contraindications to laparoscopic colectomy but should be taken into consideration especially by inexperienced practitioners [36]. Advanced age may also be considered an independent risk factor for complications [37].

The choice of an airway device is the initial step in anesthesia management. Endotracheal intubation is a reliable choice as it ensures airway protection against aspiration and control of ventilation to avoid hyper- or hypocapnia. The role of other airway access devices, such as laryngeal mask airway (LMA), has not yet been well established. There are valid concerns regarding the risk of gastric content aspiration and suboptimal ventilation [38]. The use of newer generation LMAs may be of use in brief laparoscopic procedures (e.g., cholecystectomy) but as of now there does not seem to be a place for them in laparoscopic colorectal surgery [39].

General anesthesia is the only safe and acceptable option in these types of procedures. Regional anesthesia techniques such as spinal anesthesia have been proven to be successful in shorter procedures and there have been reports of successful implementation in laparoscopic colectomy [40]. However, concerns regarding adequate levels of anesthesia (especially in subcostal areas), patient discomfort due to positioning and the likelihood of pneumoperitoneum-induced hypercapnia render this approach problematic.

Induction and maintenance of anesthesia can be accomplished with either intravenous or inhalation agents or a combination of the two, depending on patient-specific factors and personal preference. In most cases, IV agents provide shorter induction times and are usually preferred for induction in adults. Inhalation agents usually require prolonged ventilation during induction which can lead to gastric and bowel distention which in turn can increase the risk of perforation during Verres needle insertion. However, sevoflurane has a relative short time period for the onset of loss of conscientiousness and is therefore an attractive alternative [41]. The use of nitrous oxide (N2O) in laparoscopic colorectal surgery can be troublesome. N_2O has a propensity to accumulate in hollow cavities in the body, including the intestine, and is avoided during induction and maintenance of anesthesia in laparoscopic surgery [42].

Neuromuscular blockade is necessary for manipulation in the abdominal cavity. There is no consensus on the optimal depth of neuromuscular blockade. For instance, deep blockade has been associated with fewer abrupt increases in IAP when performing laparoscopic colorectal surgery but quality data to support its routine use are lacking [43, 44].

Ventilation strategies have to be appropriately adjusted to accommodate changes in respiratory mechanics during pneumoperitoneum. Volume-controlled ventilation ensures the delivery of a preset tidal volume but in the case of pneumoperitoneum it carries an increased risk of barotrauma due to increases in airway pressure. Pressure-controlled ventilation reduces the risk associated with increased airway pressures and has been documented to improve lung compliance [45]. Nonetheless, it is still unclear if this type of ventilation is associated with improved arterial oxygenation especially in the steep Trendelenburg position and it should be noted that fluctuations in IAP can influence minute ventilation in this setting [46].

Positive end-expiratory pressure (PEEP) can also be adjusted in order to avoid atelectasis induced by increases in intrathoracic pressure and therefore improve arterial oxygenation. A PEEP of 5–10 mmHg in most cases can be safely employed [47]. Caution is advised in patients with severe cardiac dysfunction. The cumulative effects of increased IAP and PEEP can have deleterious hemodynamic effects.

Fluid management is another concern that needs to be addressed in the operating theater. Liberal IV fluid administration has been associated both in laparoscopic and in open colorectal surgery with an increased incidence of complications, including anastomosis leakage possibly due to bowl wall edema. Prudent and restrictive administration of fluids is warranted guided by intraoperative monitoring of hemo-dynamic status [48]. In addition, steep Trendelenburg position can compound the effects of fluid overload and result in facial and neck edema. Unfortunately, moni-toring of hemodynamic status can be challenging in laparoscopic surgery. As previ-ously mentioned, increased IAP can have a substantial effect on hemodynamic parameters thus rendering measurements such as CVP, arterial blood pressure, and urine output unreliable for optimal management. Newer technologies such as pulse pressure contour analysis have offered additional tools in the intraoperative setting but their utility in laparoscopic colorectal surgery has not been fully established [49]. Transesophageal echocardiography has been proposed as a reliable, minimally invasive technique but requires expertise and availability [48, 49]. In our experi-ence, good communication between the anesthesiologist and surgical team is just as important as traditional monitoring and adoption of newer technologies. The sur-geon needs to inform of unexpected blood loss and potential prolongation of opera-tive time. In most cases, the combination of all the aforementioned is sufficient for optimal fluid management.

Active thermoregulation should not be neglected and should be performed in laparoscopic as in open colorectal surgery, as the reduced environmental exposure of the abdominal cavity during laparoscopic surgery does not compensate for the marked effects of anesthesia on temperature [50]. Patients should receive adequate airway humidification and protection against unintentional hypothermia, due to the potential for a longer duration of the procedure.

9.7 Pain Management

One of the most salient advantages of laparoscopic surgery is the avoidance of large incisions on the abdominal wall and excessive manipulation of abdominal viscera. This results in mitigated trauma to the visceral and parietal peritoneum and there-fore less irritation of the nerve endings that transmit nocuous stimuli. However, distention of the abdominal wall, entrapment of CO_2 in anatomical compartments, and port site trauma can lead to patient discomfort and need for meticulous pain management.

Enhanced recovery after surgery (ERAS) protocols have been established in an attempt to reduce healthcare costs, improve clinical outcomes, and enhance patient satisfaction. Laparoscopic surgery and targeted pain management strategies are main pillars of this approach. One of the main goals is to minimize the administration of opioids in the postoperative setting. Opioids have been a mainstay of analgesia following major surgery. However, one of their main side effects is the delay in resumption of normal bowel function which can considerably increase the length of hospital stay especially in colorectal surgery. Therefore, attempts are made for a multimodal approach that avoids unnecessary use of narcotics.

Epidural analgesia is a well-established and invaluable adjunct in open colorectal surgery for pain management [51]. A mid-thoracic epidural catheter is usually placed in these circumstances in order to achieve adequate analgesia. This approach has been tested in laparoscopic colorectal surgery with mixed results [52]. There seem to be modest benefits in pain management which are accompanied by longer lengths of stay. In our view, any putative benefits are probably minimal at best and therefore we do not recommend epidural catheterization in laparoscopic colorectal surgery.

Other regional anesthesia modalities which have been tested, include transversus abdominis plane (TAP) blocks. In this technique, under ultrasound guidance, the space between the internal oblique muscle and transversus abdominis muscle is infiltrated with a preparation of a long-lasting local anesthetic agent such as ropivacaine or bupivacaine. In hand-assisted laparoscopic colectomy, where a more extensive incision is made, a TAP block may provide significant analgesia. However, despite the fact that systemic analysis of the data indicates that there may be benefits in reducing pain during patient mobilization, there does not seem to be enough quality evidence to support the routine use of TAP blocks in laparoscopic colorectal surgery [53]. In our opinion, the use of these regional anesthesia modalities cancel out some of the benefits of laparoscopic surgery and similar results can be obtained by less time-consuming techniques.

Infiltration of the port insertion sites with local anesthetics is a simple option for the limitation of pain in the immediate postoperative period. As in the case of TAP blocks, long-acting local anesthetics are preferred. Local wound infiltration is a relatively cheap and fast pain control method without any significant contraindications. This method may be especially useful if abdominal drains are placed, which can irritate the abdominal wall at their exit site.

Combined use of acetaminophen and cyclooxygenase 2 (COX-2) inhibitors is a reasonable first-line analgesic regimen. Synthetic opioids such as tramadol, which have a mild effect on intestinal mobility, can be added in situations where more aggressive approaches are necessary. In rare cases, where these options fail to provide adequate pain control, opioids can be added.

9.8   Conclusion

Laparoscopic colorectal surgery has been replacing open procedures and has become the standard of care. Pneumoperitoneum and the associated increases in intra-abdominal pressure create hemodynamic and respiratory changes that are not observed during traditional open abdominal surgery, and the anesthesia team has to be well versed in these alterations of physiology. There are transient effects that influence cardiac, pulmonary, and renal function amongst other systems. Decades of research have not shown adverse outcomes in otherwise healthy individuals. In the past, patients with considerably comorbidities such as cardiovascular disease and COPD were not considered candidates for prolonged laparoscopic procedures. A better understanding of the physiological implications of laparoscopy has permitted for laparoscopic colorectal surgery to be performed with safety in individuals previously considered to be high risk.

Anesthesia management has been tailored accordingly to meet the demands of increased intra-abdominal pressure and the potential for hypercapnia. Respiratory settings are adjusted as to ensure adequate oxygenation and at the same time to protect from inadvertent barotrauma. There are no significant differences compared to anesthesia management in traditional colorectal surgery during induction or maintenance of anesthesia. The same basic principles regarding anesthesia agents and IV fluid management apply.

In the postoperative setting, pain management is usually less demanding. Patients do not require regional anesthesia modalities such as epidural catheterization. The use of opioids is usually not necessary. Greater levels of patient comfort lead to early ambulation, faster resumption of normal intestinal motility, and subsequently shorter lengths of hospital stay.

References

1. O'Malley C, Cunningham AJ. Physiologic changes during laparoscopy. Anesthesiol Clin North Am. 2001;19:1–19.
2. Cowman S, Hayden P. Anaesthesia for laparoscopic surgery. Continuing Educ Anaesthesia Crit Care Pain. 2011;11:177–80.
3. Tekelioglu UY, Erdem A, Demirhan A, et al. The prolonged effect of pneumoperitoneum on cardiac autonomic functions during laparoscopic surgery; are we aware? Eur Rev Med Pharmacol Sci. 2013;17:895 902.
4. Kadam PG, Marda M, Shah VR. Carbon dioxide absorption during laparoscopic donor nephrectomy: a comparison between retroperitoneal and transperitoneal approaches. Transplant Proc. 2008;40:1119–21.
5. Phong SV, Koh LK. Anaesthesia for robotic-assisted radical prostatectomy: considerations for laparoscopy in the Trendelenburg position. Anaesth Intensive Care. 2007;35:281–5.
6. Atkinson TM, Giraud GD, Togioka BM, Jones DB, Cigarroa JE. Cardiovascular and ventilatory consequences of laparoscopic surgery. Circulation. 2017;135:700–10.
7. Ishizaki Y, Bandai Y, Shimomura K, Abe H, Ohtomo Y, Idezuki Y. Safe intraabdominal pressure of carbon dioxide pneumoperitoneum during laparoscopic surgery. Surgery. 1993;114:549–54.
8. Meininger D, Westphal K, Bremerich DH, et al. Effects of posture and prolonged pneumoperitoneum on hemodynamic parameters during laparoscopy. World J Surg. 2008;32:1400–5.
9. Odeberg-Wernerman S. Laparoscopic surgery--effects on circulatory and respiratory physiology: an overview. Eur J Surg Suppl. 2000;(585):4–11.
10. Kitano Y, Takata M, Sasaki N, Zhang Q, Yamamoto S, Miyasaka K. Influence of increased abdominal pressure on steady-state cardiac performance. J Appl Physiol (1985). 1999;86:1651–6.

11. Neudecker J, Sauerland S, Neugebauer E, et al. The European Association for Endoscopic Surgery clinical practice guideline on the pneumoperitoneum for laparoscopic surgery. Surg Endosc. 2002;16:1121–43.
12. Gutt CN, Oniu T, Mehrabi A, et al. Circulatory and respiratory complications of carbon dioxide insufflation. Dig Surg. 2004;21:95–105.
13. Demyttenaere S, Feldman LS, Fried GM. Effect of pneumoperitoneum on renal perfusion and function: a systematic review. Surg Endosc. 2007;21:152–60.
14. Nguyen NT, Perez RV, Fleming N, Rivers R, Wolfe BM. Effect of prolonged pneumoperitoneum on intraoperative urine output during laparoscopic gastric bypass. J Am Coll Surg. 2002;195:476–83.
15. Wiesenthal JD, Fazio LM, Perks AE, et al. Effect of pneumoperitoneum on renal tissue oxygenation and blood flow in a rat model. Urology. 2011;77:1508.e9–15.
16. Dunn MD, McDougall EM. Renal physiology. Laparoscopic considerations Urol Clin North Am. 2000;27:609–14.
17. Wever KE, Bruintjes MH, Warle MC, Hooijmans CR. Renal perfusion and function during Pneumoperitoneum: a systematic review and meta-analysis of animal studies. PLoS One. 2016;11:e0163419.
18. Abassi Z, Bishara B, Karram T, Khatib S, Winaver J, Hoffman A. Adverse effects of pneumoperitoneum on renal function: involvement of the endothelin and nitric oxide systems. Am J Physiol Regul Integr Comp Physiol. 2008;294:R842–50.
19. Vasdev N, Poon AS, Gowrie-Mohan S, et al. The physiologic and anesthetic considerations in elderly patients undergoing robotic renal surgery. Rev Urol. 2014;16:1–9.
20. Seguro AC, Poli de Figueiredo LF, Shimizu MH. N- acetylcysteine (NAC) protects against acute kidney injury (AKI) following prolonged pneumoperitoneum in the rat. J Surg Res. 2012;175:312–5.
21. Schafer M, Krahenbuhl L. Effect of laparoscopy on intra- abdominal blood flow. Surgery. 2001;129:385–9.
22. Moon YJ, Jun IG, Kim KH, Kim SO, Song JG, Hwang GS. Comparison of acute kidney injury between open and laparoscopic liver resection: propensity score analysis. PLoS One. 2017;12:e0186336.
23. Kamine TH, Papavassiliou E, Schneider BE. Effect of abdominal insufflation for laparoscopy on intracranial pressure. JAMA Surg. 2014;149:380–2.
24. Smith M. Cerebral perfusion pressure. Br J Anaesth. 2015;115:488–90.
25. Robba C, Cardim D, Donnelly J, et al. Effects of pneumoperitoneum and Trendelenburg position on intracranial pressure assessed using different non- invasive methods. Br J Anaesth. 2016;117:783–91.
26. Kalmar AF, Dewaele F, Foubert L, et al. Cerebral haemodynamic physiology during steep Trendelenburg position and CO(2) pneumoperitoneum. Br J Anaesth. 2012;108:478–84.
27. Huettemann E, Terborg C, Sakka SG, Petrat G, Schier F, Reinhart K. Preserved CO(2) reactivity and increase in middle cerebral arterial blood flow velocity during laparoscopic surgery in children. Anesth Analg. 2002;94:255–8, table of contents
28. Hatipoglu S, Akbulut S, Hatipoglu F, Abdullayev R. Effect of laparoscopic abdominal surgery on splanchnic circulation: historical developments. World J Gastroenterol. 2014;20:18165–76.
29. Marana E, Scambia G, Maussier ML, et al. Neuroendocrine stress response in patients undergoing benign ovarian cyst surgery by laparoscopy, minilaparotomy, and laparotomy. J Am Assoc Gynecol Laparosc. 2003;10:159–65.
30. Riese J, Schoolmann S, Beyer A, Denzel C, Hohenberger W, Haupt W. Production of IL-6 and MCP-1 by the human peritoneum in vivo during major abdominal surgery. Shock. 2000;14:91–4.
31. Hubner M, Mantziari S, Demartines N, Pralong F, Coti-Bertrand P, Schafer M. Postoperative albumin drop is a marker for surgical stress and a predictor for clinical outcome: a pilot study. Gastroenterol Res Pract. 2016;2016:8743187.
32. Okholm C, Goetze JP, Svendsen LB, Achiam MP. Inflammatory response in laparoscopic vs. open surgery for gastric cancer. Scand J Gastroenterol. 2014;49:1027–34.

33. Biondi A, Grosso G, Mistretta A, et al. Laparoscopic vs. open approach for colorectal cancer: evolution over time of minimal invasive surgery. BMC Surg. 2013;13(Suppl 2):S12.

34. Buunen M, Gholghesaei M, Veldkamp R, Meijer DW, Bonjer HJ, Bouvy ND. Stress response to laparoscopic surgery: a review. Surg Endosc. 2004;18:1022–8.

35. Novitsky YW, Litwin DE, Callery MP. The net immunologic advantage of laparoscopic surgery. Surg Endosc. 2004;18:1411–9.

36. Pisano CW. Laparoscopy. In: Aglio LS, Urman RD, editors. Anesthesiology: clinical case reviews. Cham: Springer International Publishing; 2017. p. 247–53.

37. Scheidbach H, Schneider C, Hügel O, Yildirim C, Lippert H, Köckerling F. Laparoscopic surgery in the old patient: do indications and outcomes differ? Langenbeck's Arch Surg. 2005;390:328–32.

38. Belena JM, Ochoa EJ, Nunez M, Gilsanz C, Vidal A. Role of laryngeal mask airway in laparoscopic cholecystectomy. World J Gastrointest Surg. 2015;7:319–25.

39. Timmermann A, Bergner UA, Russo SG. Laryngeal mask airway indications: new frontiers for second-generation supraglottic airways. Curr Opin Anesthesiol. 2015;28:717–26.

40. Sinha R, Gurwara AK, Gupta SC. Laparoscopic surgery using spinal anesthesia. JSLS. 2008;12:133–8.

41. Boonmak P, Boonmak S, Pattanittum P. High initial concentration versus low initial concentration sevoflurane for inhalational induction of anaesthesia. Cochrane Database Syst Rev 2016;(6):CD006837.

42. Akca O, Lenhardt R, Fleischmann E, et al. Nitrous oxide increases the incidence of bowel distension in patients undergoing elective colon resection. Acta Anaesthesiol Scand. 2004;48:894–8.

43. Koo BW, Oh AY, Na HS, et al. Effects of depth of neuromuscular block on surgical conditions during laparoscopic colorectal surgery: a randomised controlled trial. Anaesthesia. 2018;73:1090–6.

44. Park SK, Son YG, Yoo S, Lim T, Kim WH, Kim JT. Deep vs. moderate neuromuscular blockade during laparoscopic surgery: a systematic review and meta- analysis. Eur J Anaesthesiol. 2018;35:867–75.

45. Ogurlu M, Kucuk M, Bilgin F, et al. Pressure-controlled vs volume-controlled ventilation during laparoscopic gynecologic surgery. J Minim Invasive Gynecol. 2010;17:295–300.

46. Choi EM, Na S, Choi SH, An J, Rha KH, Oh YJ. Comparison of volume-controlled and pressure- controlled ventilation in steep Trendelenburg position for robot-assisted laparoscopic radical prostatectomy. J Clin Anesth. 2011;23:183–8.

47. Meininger D, Byhahn C, Mierdl S, Westphal K, Zwissler B. Positive end-expiratory pressure improves arterial oxygenation during prolonged pneumoperitoneum. Acta Anaesthesiol Scand. 2005;49:778–83.

48. Alfonsi P, Slim K, Chauvin M, et al. French guidelines for enhanced recovery after elective colorectal surgery. J Visc Surg. 2014;151:65–79.

49. Concha MR, Mertz VF, Cortinez LI, Gonzalez KA, Butte JM. Pulse contour analysis and transesophageal echocardiography: a comparison of measurements of cardiac output during laparoscopic colon surgery. Anesth Analg. 2009;109:114–8.

50. Jacobs VR, Morrison JE Jr, Mettler L, Mundhenke C, Jonat W. Measurement of CO_2 hypothermia during laparoscopy and pelviscopy: how cold it gets and how to prevent it. J Am Assoc Gynecol Laparosc. 1999;6:289–95.

51. Werawatganon T, Charuluxanun S. Patient controlled intravenous opioid analgesia versus continuous epidural analgesia for pain after intra-abdominal surgery. Cochrane Database Syst Rev 2005;(1):CD004088.

52. Joshi GP, Schug SA, Kehlet H. Procedure-specific pain management and outcome strategies. Best Pract Res Clin Anaesthesiol. 2014;28:191–201.

53. Oh TK, Lee S-J, Do S-H, Song I-A. Transversus abdominis plane block using a short-acting local anesthetic for postoperative pain after laparoscopic colorectal surgery: a systematic review and meta-analysis. Surg Endosc. 2018;32:545–52.

Acronyms

ADH	Antidiuretic hormone
CI	Cardiac index
CO_2	Carbon dioxide
COPD	Chronic obstructive pulmonary disease
CPP	Cerebral perfusion pressure
CSF	Cerebrospinal fluid
CVP	Central venous pressure
ECG	Electrocardiogram
ET-1	Endothelin 1
$ETCO_2$ or $etCO_2$	End tidal carbon dioxide
FRC	Functional residual capacity
GFR	Glomerular filtration rate
IAP	Intra-abdominal pressure
ICP	Intracranial pressure
IL (1,6,8)	Interleukin (1,6,8)
IPPV	Intermittent positive pressure ventilation
NIBP	Noninvasive blood pressure
$PaCO_2$	Arterial partial pressure of carbon dioxide
PCWP	Pulmonary capillaries wedge pressure
PEEP	Positive end expiratory pressure
RBF	Renal blood flow
SVR	Systemic vascular resistance
TNF	Tumor necrosis factor
V/Q	Ventilation/perfusion ratio

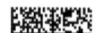